AF092458

think less,
SLEEP
MORE

Stephanie Romiszewski is a UK-based sleep expert who has helped over 10,000 patients, from Premier League footballers and high-profile CEOs to new parents and shift workers, fix their sleep. She combines academic expertize – including degrees in psychology and behavioural sleep medicine and experience within the NHS and Harvard Medical School – with deep and broad media experience across TV, radio, podcasts and social media, and has appeared on the high-profile *Diary of a CEO* with Steven Bartlett. The sleep expert in both Channel 4's *Secrets of Sleep* series and the BBC's *Insomnia and Me*, Stephanie is also the presenter of the *Sleep Better* course for BBC Maestro and one of the specialists behind the virtual insomnia clinic re:sleep. Since 2014, she has run the Sleepyhead Clinic.

www.sleepyheadclinic.co.uk

think less, SLEEP MORE

From Panic & Perfectionism to Stress-free Sleep

Stephanie Romiszewski

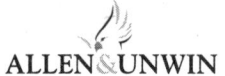

ALLEN&UNWIN

First published in trade paperback in Great Britain in 2026 by Allen & Unwin, an imprint of Atlantic Books Ltd.

Copyright © Stephanie Romiszewski, 2026

The moral right of Stephanie Romiszewski to be identified as the author of this work has been asserted by her in accordance with the Copyright, Designs and Patents Act of 1988.

All rights reserved. No part of this publication may be reproduced, stored in a retrieval system, or transmitted in any form or by any means, electronic, mechanical, photocopying, recording, or otherwise, without the prior permission of both the copyright owner and the above publisher of this book.

No part of this book may be used in any manner in the learning, training or development of generative artificial intelligence technologies (including but not limited to machine learning models and large language models (LLMs)), whether by data scraping, data mining or use in any way to create or form a part of data sets or in any other way.

All illustrations © Hannah Wilson, Quoted Visually. Used with permission and thanks.

Every effort has been made to trace or contact all copyright holders. The publishers will be pleased to make good any omissions or rectify any mistakes brought to their attention at the earliest opportunity.

10 9 8 7 6 5 4 3

A CIP catalogue record for this book is available from the British Library.

Trade Paperback ISBN: 978 1 80546 455 6
E-book ISBN: 978 1 80546 456 3

Printed and bound by CPI Group (UK) Ltd, Croydon CR0 4YY

Allen & Unwin
An imprint of Atlantic Books Ltd
Ormond House
26–27 Boswell Street
London
WC1N 3JZ

www.atlantic-books.co.uk

Product safety EU representative: Authorised Rep Compliance Ltd., Ground Floor, 71 Lower Baggot Street, Dublin, D02 P593, Ireland. www.arccompliance.com

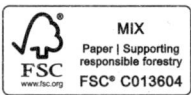

For Ander:
You were with me the whole way.
This is for your generation.

Contents

Prologue ix

Introduction 1

Part 1: The Two Conflicting Stories of Sleep   **11**

Chapter 1   We Didn't Always Obsess Like This: How We Naturally Sleep   13

Chapter 2   How We Got So Weird About Sleep – and Why It's Making Us Sleep Worse   57

Part 2: Sleep 2.0: Your New Sleep Operating System   **73**

Chapter 3   Sleep Sensitivity: The Dripping Tap, the Ticking Clock...   75

Chapter 4   Why Your Morning Matters More Than Your Evening   87

Chapter 5   Tired But Wired: Meet the Sleep Anxiety Gremlins   123

Chapter 6   Sleep Isn't a Bank: Stop Making Deposits   147

Chapter 7   The Sleep Tools Trap: When Help Stops Helping   161

Part 3: The Joy of Imperfect Sleep — 219

Chapter 8	The Definition of a Good Sleeper	223
Chapter 9	Stop Blaming Sleep for Everything	241
Chapter 10	Free Yourself from Sleep Perfectionism: How to Be AWAKE	249
Conclusion	Viva La Sleep Revolution!	261
Appendix	Sleep Disorders: When You Need More Support	273

Notes and References — 291

Acknowledgements — 309

Prologue

Amaya falls asleep easily at 11 p.m. She wakes at 2 a.m., stays awake for thirty minutes, then drifts back to sleep until 6 a.m. Luca sleeps through most of the night, but wakes briefly at 4 a.m. and again at 5 a.m., lying awake for ten minutes before slipping back into sleep. Emma tosses and turns intermittently during the first half of the night, but falls back to sleep after each brief wake-up. Mark takes forty-five minutes to fall asleep after a particularly hectic day, then wakes at 3 a.m., checks the time and, after twenty minutes, drifts back off. These nights of sleep are different, but they're all completely normal.

Then there's Clara. She stays up late, drinks espresso at 9 p.m. and eats a large meal right before bed. She falls asleep easily and sleeps straight through the night.

The way we've been taught to think about sleep is often completely wrong. We've been sold the idea that perfect sleep requires perfect conditions. But, in reality, there's a huge range of normal, and doing the 'wrong' things doesn't automatically mean bad sleep.

We will step away from this type of thinking now, and explore a new way forward – one with outcomes that will not only improve sleep through the ups and downs of life, but take away the constant pressure and replace it with feeling good about ourselves.

Introduction

You know that feeling. The alarm goes off. Your body is cemented to the bed. You hit snooze, maybe twice, maybe three times, because getting up feels like trying to lift a 450-kg weight. And then, the dread creeps in. *Today is going to be a struggle.*

You think back to last night – another battle with sleep, another night of tossing, turning, watching the clock and calculating (and recalculating) the hours left until morning. And now, here you are, dragging yourself through the day in a fog, barely present, just about coping. *If I could just fix my sleep,* you think. *If I could just sleep normally, everything would be easier.*

Imagine starting your day without having to snooze your alarm three times before you can muster any kind of energy to just get up; without that overwhelming feeling of dread; without the weight of knowing that today will feel like a struggle because of another restless night. Or think about going through a full day, focused and energized, without the constant brain fog or that crushing fatigue that makes every task feel twice as hard. These aren't just dreams – they're real changes you can make, and I'm here to show you how.

This book will challenge some of the most common assumptions you've heard about sleep. You might think the secret to better sleep lies in perfecting your evening routine, but what if I told you that your morning habits may have a bigger impact than anything you do before bed? Perhaps you've been told that achieving deep sleep is about strict rituals, supplements and tracking every minute spent in REM. Yet, despite your best efforts, you still find yourself staring at the ceiling, more awake than before. Do you spend time calculating and worrying about how much sleep you will get if you fall asleep right now? Do you tell yourself that if you don't get it, tomorrow will be ruined? If any of this sounds familiar, you're not alone. And, more importantly, there's a way out.

Sleep Anxiety and the Search for 'Perfect' Sleep

For the past two decades, I've been in the business of researching, and then fixing, broken sleep. Not by citing endless studies, but by seeing what actually works for people who struggle, in real life, to get the sleep they need – to resolve really severe and often complex sleep disorders, for good. From an inability to get to sleep, lying in bed for hours and sometimes all night, to people who wake up and just can't maintain the sleep... and everything in between and for all sorts of reasons – from pain to stress to parenting to menopause – we would call these issues 'insomnias'. I've also worked with hypersomnias (disorders of sleepiness such as sleep apnoea and narcolepsy) and parasomnias (from sleepwalking and sleep talking to sleep sex) – and while these are less common than insomnia and behave very differently, it has given me the best education in what 'normal' sleep really looks like.

But something has changed. My clinics used to be filled with people suffering from medical sleep disorders. Now, more and more, I see people whose biggest issue isn't a clinical disorder – it's fear. They come in with reams of data and measurements from their sleep trackers (which, ironically, can lead to chronic insomnia sleep disorder), convinced that one bad night has ruined their health forever. They don't just struggle with sleep; they panic about it. And it's causing problems.

If you've ever felt like you're one bad night away from disaster, you're not imagining things. Sleep has been dragged into the spotlight over recent years and, while it's good that people are paying attention to their health, there has been an unintended side effect: sleep anxiety. The more we've been told to optimize, track and protect our sleep, the more we've started to fear it, treating it as something fragile and elusive rather than a natural process. Suddenly, sleep – one of the most natural and uncontrollable processes – has become a source of stress, something to calculate, measure and control.

But sleep was never meant to be this complicated. You are not broken. You are not going to 'lose' your ability to sleep. You do not have to earn rest through perfect conditions. Sleep is a shared thread that connects us all, no matter who we are. It is the great equalizer. Whether you're a nurse working night shifts, a firefighter on call or a new parent waking at odd hours, sleep is a universal human rhythm. If something so natural and essential can function across all kinds of lives and situations, from astronauts to artists, then surely it does not need to be micromanaged, feared or controlled into submission.

Yet, the headlines tell a different story. We are constantly warned that sleeping fewer than six hours is a death sentence, that bad sleep is shaving years off our lives or that our future health is doomed if we don't hit the perfect sleep scores. But these claims often overlook context – who was studied, how sleep was measured and what the long-term outcomes really mean. Take the often-cited Penn State study, which looked at a very specific group: people with chronic insomnia *and* objectively measured short sleep duration. Yes, it showed that these individuals, those with consistently broken, unrefreshing sleep, had worse health outcomes. But this group is far from typical and, most importantly, these patterns can often be improved. In fact, people who sleep fewer hours but feel refreshed and function well don't show the same risks at all.

This book is not here to throw more statistics at you, make you feel like you're in a laboratory or add to the fear-mongering that makes sleep feel like a test you're constantly failing. Quite the opposite. It is here to liberate you from the anxiety that this kind of 'perfect sleep' thinking has caused.

There's no 'one-size-fits-all' when it comes to sleep, and we don't need to be perfect in order to get good sleep. Sleep should be manageable, realistic and, above all, natural. And this is why my approach here – one developed through working with over 10,000 clients who've faced the full range of sleep issues – doesn't rely on forcing perfect sleep hygiene or setting up countless bedtime rituals, supplements and potions like an Olympic sleep athlete constantly striving for that extra 1–2 per cent. I know these people exist – and good for them! But if you can't get sleep right in the first place, this attitude won't help you. Instead, it's about easing that relentless pressure to 'fix' sleep, while taking care of some core fundamental aspects of sleep – but this isn't an endless list; it's quite simple once you know how. If you understand sleep enough, you will be able to let go of the need to perfect and control it.

I thought carefully about writing this book, but then I realized something – if I don't say this, who will? If I don't tell you that you are not broken, that your body already knows how to sleep and that you don't need to control it so tightly, then how else will you know? Spending my entire career fixing sleep disorders, interacting with clients after their sleep has gone awry, is not going to suffice – I think we sleep specialists need to be doing a better job of presenting sleep in a more balanced way, to the general population, to avoid them getting chronic sleep problems in the first place.

I promise, I am a fairly average human being. My life is not so fancy or so void of stress and normal life stuff that it's 'easy' for me to keep my sleep perfect. In fact, my sleep is not perfect, because that is literally impossible (and even attempting to make it possible means making so many sacrifices I am genuinely not interested, thank you!). The reason I never worry about sleep is not because I've hacked my way to this so-called perfection – it's because I know sleep doesn't require that.

This book is my way of handing that knowledge to you.

My experience and approach are inherently biased. After all, I've spent years as a clinician, working specifically to help people untangle themselves from the traps of chronic sleep issues, insomnia and anxiety around sleep. But I'd argue that this is exactly why I can offer you something different from what's out there right now. And it just so happens that it is in line with the science as well.

Let's talk about this 'sleep epidemic' everyone's panicking about. Yes, insomnia rates are climbing (according to one of the most recent analyses, we are currently between 10 and 30 per cent of the global population, depending on insomnia type) and sleep issues seem to be on the rise too, but I think much of this has been fuelled by misinformation. We've become anxious about sleep to the point of obsession, worrying about every aspect – from sleep stages to gadgets and routines that supposedly guarantee a better night's rest. What started as a focus on sleep health has spiralled into a fear-driven fixation that keeps people counting hours and tracking every movement instead of simply resting. And guess what – sleep did in fact exist before all this.

My hope is that this book can help you find a new, more balanced approach. We're not here to 'win' at sleep or hit some magic sleep score. Instead, I'll offer you an alternative: do less and allow sleep to become a natural ally rather than a source of fear. My philosophy is simple – sleep isn't the problem; it's the way we approach it that's making things harder than they need to be.

Yes, there is practical guidance here – I am not just about to tell you to 'accept' truly broken sleep; it does not have to be that way. I'll give you strategies that I've seen work time and again with clients who have struggled deeply with sleep. But we're going to keep things simple and realistic. We'll take on some of the myths that fuel sleep anxiety, talk about why sleep isn't something you need to micromanage and figure out how to step back from the endless chase for perfect sleep.

If you're tired of feeling like sleep is something you're

Sleep was never meant to be something you work for.

constantly fighting, you're in the right place. By the end of this book, you'll have a completely different relationship with sleep. You will no longer be a slave to sleep scores or nightly calculations and you will have the confidence to rest without fear. Sleep was never meant to be something you work for. It was meant to be something you *let happen*. Let's take it back.

One final note: this is not the treatment for chronic insomnia or any other medical sleep disorder, and while every insomnia patient of mine will go through these steps to start with to help unravel the problem, when things become as serious as a major sleep disorder, we need to make sure we get support from medical professionals and evidence-based treatments. I've spent much of my career building these types of treatments and will spend some time in the appendix helping you to understand if and when you might need to take some next steps, and what they might be. One thing is for sure, though, if you can absorb this book in the way I have designed it, you will either dramatically reduce your risk of ever getting chronic insomnia and have good sleep for most of your life, or you will be part way to treating it for good.

Think of this book as your new philosophy towards good sleep. Let's begin.

PART 1

THE TWO CONFLICTING STORIES OF SLEEP

CHAPTER 1

We Didn't Always Obsess Like This: How We Naturally Sleep

Historically, humans did not obsess over sleep the way we do today. We know this through historical accounts, anthropological evidence and the relative absence of cultural concern about sleep.

Cave people weren't lying awake, anxiously counting how many mammoth-free REM cycles they were getting. Their biggest sleep concern was whether they'd wake up inside a predator's stomach. Medieval peasants didn't check their sundials in a panic, worrying that their biphasic sleep pattern was 'suboptimal'. They got up in the middle of the night, had a snack, chatted with their spouse and went back to sleep without a second thought. Even the Victorians – who had rules for everything from table manners to how one should properly mourn a dead parrot – weren't tracking their sleep debt in a leather-bound journal.

Sleep has been seen as a natural and unforced part of life for most of human history, shaped by the planet's natural rhythms. Before artificial light and modern schedules, people relied on natural light cues to regulate sleep and wakefulness. The sun's rising and setting dictated daily patterns, with daylight signalling activity and darkness signalling rest. People simply responded to these cues without analysing or controlling their sleep. And did they sleep worse? Not necessarily. In fact, they may have slept with fewer barriers than we do today. Historical and anthropological evidence suggests that many pre-industrial societies slept in alignment with natural light, had flexible sleep patterns and lacked the chronic sleep anxiety we see today. Without artificial light, rigid work schedules or constant stimulation, sleep was allowed to unfold naturally.

In medieval Europe, for example, records describe this biphasic sleep, where people naturally slept in two phases: a 'first sleep' early in the night, followed by a period of wakefulness used sometimes for prayer, socializing or quiet reflection, before returning to a 'second sleep'. This was not something they tried to fix – it was just normal. In texts, diaries and literature from this time, we find little mention of sleep concerns the way we do now, or widespread anxiety about rest quality.

Anthropological studies of modern hunter-gatherer societies, such as the Hadza in Tanzania and the San in Namibia, offer further insight into how humans likely slept before industrialization. These communities still follow natural patterns, rising with the sun and sleeping after sunset, with sleep varying seasonally and flexibly depending on temperature, activity and the group's needs. And, crucially, they do not report sleep anxiety. Sleep happens naturally, without the pressure to track, optimize or perfect it.

So, what changed?

What changed was industrialization. The invention of mechanical clocks and artificial light disrupted the natural alignment between sleep and the environment. With longer working hours and an emphasis on productivity, sleep began to be seen as inconvenient – something that got in the way of progress. By the twentieth century, sleep wasn't just a function of biology, it had become a problem to manage. Advances in sleep science, while groundbreaking, also created new anxieties. The more we measured sleep, the more we worried about it. Tools to compare sleep introduced expectations of a 'perfect' eight hours and, when people fell short, they began to feel inadequate (as demonstrated by researcher Kohler in his study on sleep tracking, and many others).

These anxieties have only grown in recent years with the rise of sleep trackers, apps and endless 'sleep hacks'. While these tools were designed to help, they've often made sleep feel like something to constantly monitor and perfect – turning a natural, adaptable process into yet another area of life to optimize. Ironically, this has made sleep worse for many people, not better.

But this brings us to a crucial question: how does sleep actually work? If sleep is adaptable, can't we 'hack' it? And since we live in a world that's different from the one our ancestors lived in, what does that mean for us today?

If we're going to understand sleep properly, we have to start with the two main forces that control it: sleep drive and circadian rhythm. These two systems work together to determine when you sleep, how long you sleep and how well you sleep.

Sleep Drive: Your Internal Sleep Pressure

Sleep drive, also known as the homeostatic process, is what makes you feel sleepy the longer you stay awake. The moment you wake up, sleep pressure starts building in your brain, thanks to a chemical called adenosine. This pressure grows steadily throughout the day until you can't resist sleep anymore. Then you sleep, the pressure goes down and you find yourself awake to start the whole process again.

It's kind of ironic – the only way to build sleep pressure is by being awake. And yet, modern society has made 'spending time awake' feel like a failure. It's like we have

Sleep has been turned from a natural, adaptable process into yet another area of life to optimize.

forgotten that it's simply part of the natural cycle that leads to sleep.

Think of sleep drive like a phone battery. You can't use your phone without charging it, and you can't sleep if you haven't spent enough time awake. But, unlike a phone battery, your body doesn't need you to micromanage it – it knows how to reset itself. Phone batteries also become very unpredictable when we start charging them sporadically and, over time, that battery can become weak. This is exactly what happens to your sleep drive, and in later chapters we will explore how we muck this process up and how we can make it better again.

Circadian Rhythm: Your Internal Body Clock

If sleep drive determines *how tired* you are, circadian rhythm determines *when you feel ready for sleep*. This is your internal clock, running on a roughly twenty-four-hour cycle, influenced primarily by light. It's like the master timekeeper of your body, regulating more than just sleep – your digestion, mood and even body temperature follow this cycle too.

It's amazing, really – light means so much to us. We are more like plants than we think! We evolved on this particular planet, which, due to its rotation and light–dark cycles, runs on a roughly twenty-four-hour day. This is why our bodies don't just follow an internal schedule – they sync to the environment.

Before artificial lighting (industrialization interfering again), humans' circadian rhythms were naturally aligned with the sun. Sunlight triggered wakefulness and darkness signalled melatonin production (our 'sleepy' hormone), preparing us for rest. But this wasn't rigid – because the Earth's rotation brings seasonal shifts in daylight, human sleep patterns have always had some level of flexibility.

In some pre-industrial societies living at extreme latitudes, people adapted their sleep in fascinating ways. During long winter nights, what's known as 'segmented sleep' was common – people would sleep for a few hours, wake naturally for one or two, then return to sleep, and this wakeful period wasn't considered unusual.

There's less formal documentation for how people coped during long summer days, but writer Jessa Gamble (in *The Siesta and the Midnight Sun*) describes anthropological observations from circumpolar cultures – such as the Sámi people in Scandinavia or Indigenous Alaskan groups – suggesting that sleep often became more fragmented or delayed during periods of constant daylight. People adapted by resting during the dimmest parts of the 'night' or by relying on environmental and social cues, like going indoors or darkening their spaces, to signal rest time. Crucially, this wasn't treated as a disorder – it was simply a practical response to environmental extremes.

This brings up an interesting question: in places with these extreme light conditions today, do people sleep more or less? Surprisingly, modern data shows that national averages for sleep duration don't vary as wildly as you'd expect. Why? Because artificial lighting, cultural routines, work schedules and social norms often override natural light cues. In essence, while our internal clocks are *meant* to sync with the sun, our lifestyles often pull them in different directions. That's why supporting your circadian rhythm intentionally – especially through morning light exposure – matters now more than ever (more on this in Part 2).

And here's the key point: sleep consistency matters, but sleep perfection does not. In fact, being super rigid with your sleep schedule can backfire. After all, human sleep has always had to adapt to the environment. Flexibility isn't a flaw in your sleep – it's a feature.

How These Two Systems Work Together

When sleep drive and circadian rhythm are aligned, sleep feels effortless. You get tired at night, fall asleep quickly and wake up ready to be awake. But when they're out of sync – because of artificial light, shift work, jet lag or bad sleep habits – sleep can feel impossible, even if you feel exhausted, or, if you can achieve it, it is light and broken.

This is often when someone pipes up and says, 'Let's go back to sleeping with natural time cues then,' which

Two sleep mechanisms

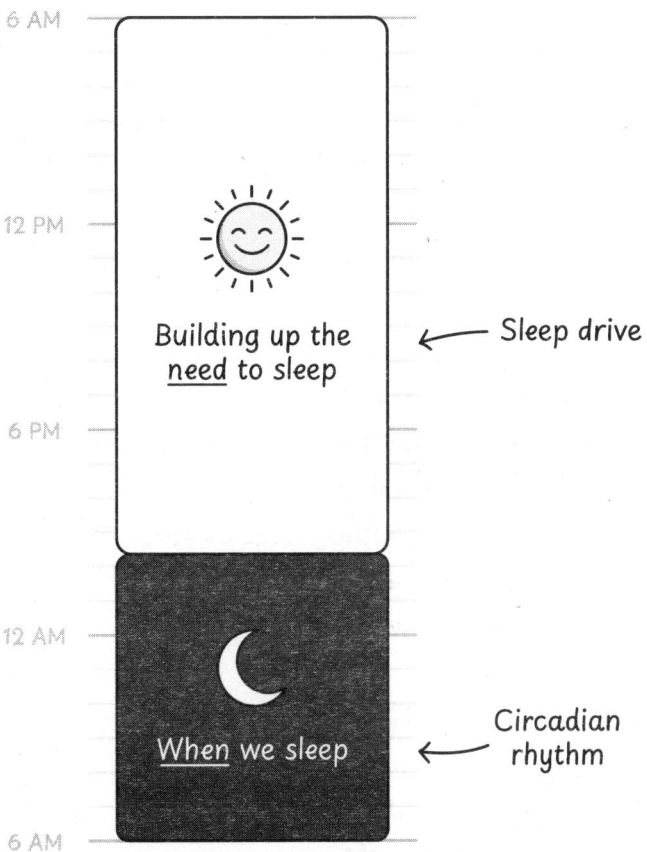

would involve things like getting up with the sun, whenever it rises. But while understanding the mechanisms of sleep and how we used to do it is helpful, we still live in the new modern world and it's not going anywhere. We can't have one foot in the past while still wanting artificial light, a schedule that fits work and all our idealistic lifestyle preferences – unless you're a multi-millionaire, of course, and have complete control over literally every part of your life to influence your sleep or you live in nature with no human-like interferences, such as a job or technology or even a social life. It's just not that simple.

So, what can we do instead? To understand why this is a flawed approach, we first need to break down how sleep actually works after darkness falls, sleep pressure (adenosine) has been built and that lovely sleepy hormone (melatonin) is present – and why every stage matters, even the ones we barely notice.

What's Actually Happening When You Sleep?

Most people think of sleep as one continuous block of rest. In reality, sleep is a series of repeating cycles, each lasting 90–110 minutes or so. A full night consists of four to five of these cycles, and each stage within them serves a different, crucial function. Don't be fooled into thinking these cycles should remain uninterrupted either – they can naturally break and shift throughout the night. Let me explain.

Stage 1
(N1 – light sleep, ~5 per cent of total sleep time)

The most important thing to note here is that sleep doesn't happen the moment your head hits the pillow – and it's not supposed to. The average person takes between fifteen and twenty minutes to fall asleep. That's completely normal. And then enter stage 1. This is the transition from wakefulness to sleep, a fragile and fleeting stage. You drift in and out, sometimes feeling like you're still awake. This is when:

- Your muscles relax, but not always smoothly. This is when 'hypnic jerks' (that sudden falling sensation) happen. The brain misfires during this transition, briefly waking you up. It's completely normal to happen every now and then. I personally seem to be falling off a kerb or out of a plane in my dreams when this happens!
- Your brain activity slows, but it's still responsive to external noise. If someone calls your name, you'll probably wake up thinking you were never asleep at all. (Spoiler: you were.)
- Your senses remain semi-active, which is why a slight movement or a distant noise can still wake you. It also means you can have conscious thought, even though you aren't awake. This

is one of the things that makes us so useless at figuring out how much time we spend asleep (not that this matters as much as we think it does – but we do seem to spend an awful lot of time guessing). We experience these lighter stages multiple times in the night without realizing we've been sleeping at all.

Stage 2
(N2 – stable sleep, ~50 per cent of total sleep time)

Stage 2 is often underrated, yet we spend more time here than in any other stage – that's what's supposed to happen, contrary to many sleep tracking apps out there that like to overemphasize other stages. It acts as a bridge between light and deep sleep.

In stage 2:

- Your brain starts doing a major clean-up, deciding what's worth remembering and what can be forgotten. Short bursts of brain activity, called sleep spindles, appear. These are linked to learning, memory and problem-solving.
- Your body temperature drops, which is why people instinctively reach for blankets during this stage.

Most sleep trackers ignore stage 2 because it's not 'deep sleep' or 'REM', but, without it, your brain would struggle to transition between them. It's the glue that holds everything together.

Stage 3
(N3 – deep sleep, ~15–25 per cent of total sleep time)

Deep sleep is what makes you feel physically restored. It's when your body rebuilds itself, focusing on repair and recovery:

- Tissues repair, muscles grow and your immune system gets stronger.
- Your brain flushes out waste, a process linked to long-term brain health. (Think of it like an overnight cleaning crew tidying up).

You are incredibly hard to wake from deep sleep. If someone shakes you (or if your alarm catches you in this stage), you'll feel groggy and disoriented – hello, sleep inertia (see box below).

Deep sleep is front-loaded in the first half of the night.

REM sleep
('dreaming' sleep, ~20–25 per cent of total sleep time)

People assume REM is deep sleep, but it's actually the lightest stage – your brain is as active as when you're awake; it's just different.

- Your body is paralysed to prevent you from acting out dreams – except in rare cases, like REM sleep behaviour disorder, where people actually move or, in even rarer cases, attack their partners in their sleep.
- REM is crucial for emotional processing. Ever had a terrible day and felt better after a night of sleep? That's REM helping your brain reprocess emotional events.
- Most vivid dreams happen in REM. If you remember a dream in graphic detail, you were likely pulled out of REM at just the right moment, and this is a very normal phenomenon every now and again.
- As the night progresses, REM cycles get longer. This is why the second half of your night is important. There's a common myth that 'the sleep before midnight is the most important' or that the first half of the night is more restorative than the second. This isn't true. It only feels that way because deep sleep is dominant in the first half. But you need the whole night to function well.

It's easy to misread how we feel in the morning. We tend to fixate on how long we slept or whether we got enough deep sleep, but that's only part of the picture. REM plays a huge role too, especially when we have had a tough, emotional day. Even then, it's about the overall balance of what makes up your night of sleep, versus the timing of sleep, the drive to sleep and so many other factors that have nothing to do with sleep! This is important, because when we over-focus on one aspect of sleep, it doesn't usually solve the problem.

> ### Sleep inertia
>
> That groggy, fuzzy-headed feeling you sometimes get after waking is completely normal. It's not a sign that something's gone wrong – it's just your brain taking a little time to move from sleep to full alertness, especially if you've woken from a deeper stage of sleep (which, by the way, is a sign you were getting good-quality rest).
>
> Some people feel it for just a few minutes; others feel like their head is full of sand for half an hour. That's okay. It's just part of the process. But here's the good news: you can reduce how often it happens and how long it lasts.
>
> A lot of this comes down to rhythm. When your wake time is consistent and your sleep pressure is strong (which I will teach you), your body starts to time your lighter sleep stages closer to your natural wake-up. That means you're less likely to be pulled out of deep sleep by your alarm and you wake feeling clearer, faster.

Even when sleep inertia does show up, there are ways to shake it off more quickly. Chapter 4 is all about how your mornings can power your sleep and how simple things like light, movement, food and routine can make a huge difference to how alert you feel after waking.

Feeling groggy in the morning doesn't mean you've failed at sleep. It just means your brain's still booting up. And when you give it the right rhythm, it gets faster and more reliable at doing exactly that.

Note: if, despite a consistent sleep pattern, sleep inertia seems to hit so strongly that it doesn't go away, it may be a sign of a sleep disorder or further medical issue – see the appendix for more support (page 273).

The Brilliant (and Slightly Humbling) Reality About Sleep

A lot of people believe that 'good sleep' means a solid, uninterrupted block of rest. But that's completely wrong. Even healthy sleepers wake up multiple times per night. We see this in overnight sleep studies – literally everyone wakes up. The difference? People without sleep anxiety don't notice or care when they wake up. They roll over and go back to sleep, most of the time.

So, why do we wake up? REM sleep is naturally light, so, by morning, you're one noise, movement or temperature shift away from waking up. Environmental factors – like a car outside, a partner stirring or a change in temperature – can momentarily wake you up, especially in lighter sleep stages.

Good sleep isn't about staying unconscious for eight perfect hours (more on this duration myth later); it's about your sleep being fairly restorative most of the time, even with brief awakenings.

Here's something amazing: your body is already a sleep hacker – and it doesn't need your help. When you go into sleep debt (meaning you've had too little sleep over several nights), your body doesn't necessarily make up for it by increasing total sleep time. Instead, it reallocates how much time you spend in certain sleep stages to prioritize what's missing. I'd like to point out a couple of things here: firstly, like I said before, we are really bad at estimating exactly how much sleep we have had, so this process doesn't happen when your expectations think you are sleep-deprived, but when your body *knows* you are indeed sleep-deprived. This is an important distinction because we do get very overexcited about what we think should be happening and when (which sets us up for worry and disappointment when those expectations aren't met). Secondly, when we are truly sleep-deprived, we always expect our bodies to make up the duration of sleep, when it's actually far cleverer and sometimes only readjusts what stages you need.

If you've been physically exhausted or recovering from illness, your body will increase the percentage of deep sleep – even if your total sleep time stays the same. If

We think good sleep means perfection:

But even good sleep varies:

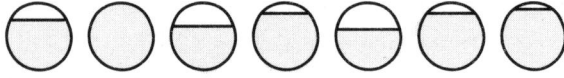

you've been emotionally drained, stressed or mentally overworked, your body will increase REM sleep, even condensing deep sleep slightly to make room for it. If you've had multiple nights of poor sleep, your sleep cycles may temporarily shift, giving you more slow-wave deep sleep early on and more REM later – even if you don't sleep longer than usual. This process is known as selective rebound – it is your brain's way of prioritizing what's most important, whether that's deep sleep for physical repair or REM sleep for emotional recovery, even without increasing total sleep time. This is why pulling an all-nighter and then sleeping for twelve hours the next night (*if* you can actually achieve this) doesn't 'reset' you. Your body doesn't simply repay sleep like a bank loan – it prioritizes the most essential recovery processes first. We will talk again about this fascinating area in Chapter 6, as, in order to look after sleep, we really need to break down our sleep debt 'eye-for-an-eye' approach more fully.

Why the military thought they could hack this (and why they were wrong)

My mum used to tell me something very interesting about my grandad's sleep when he was an officer in the Second World War. The military used to give him pills to stay awake and pills to go to sleep. Consequently, this, we believe, might have been a major contributing factor to his poor mental health in later years. That's another story, but it piqued my interest in what else they might have done to try to manipulate sleep. When researchers and military organizations realized that the body could adapt its sleep architecture, they assumed they could force this process to work more efficiently.

For decades, the military and government have tried to create 'super soldiers' who need less sleep. The goal was simple: remove 'unnecessary' sleep stages while preserving deep sleep and REM to maximize performance. Pharmaceutical approaches (for example, temazepam) successfully increased total sleep time, but soldiers weren't more alert the next day. Brain stimulation to enhance deep sleep showed promise, but had unpredictable results. Efforts to eliminate stages 1 and 2 led to disoriented, memory-impaired soldiers.

But here's the problem: we still don't fully understand why light sleep (stages 1 and 2) is so dominant. The fact that it resists being removed suggests it plays a crucial role we haven't figured out yet. When scientists tried

> to artificially extend deep sleep and REM, performance and alertness didn't improve the way they expected. Something was still missing.

Trying to micromanage sleep is like overthinking your breathing – the system already knows what it's doing and, when we overthink it, we make it worse. Your sleep has evolved over millions of years to adapt to different conditions, anticipate disruptions and prioritize what's essential. You don't need to force it – it's already adjusting for you.

Yet technology is now pushing us to do what the military failed to do – train ourselves to get 'better' sleep by forcing more deep sleep or REM while reducing other stages. If a sleep tracker tells you 'you only got 10 per cent REM last night', it implies something is wrong – even though REM naturally fluctuates night to night. Devices assign arbitrary 'sleep scores' that don't actually reflect how well-rested you feel. People wake up feeling fine, check their app, see a low score and suddenly feel exhausted.

If we can't 'hack' sleep, then what can we do? The answer isn't increasing a specific stage or forcing longer sleep – it's about improving overall sleep quality and working with the natural timing of sleep. And that's exactly what we'll cover in Part 2.

Things That Go Bump In the Night...

But I have loads of hypnic jerks, and random stuff happens in my sleep, like sleep talking and night terrors – it's exhausting! Sleep naturally fluctuates, and occasional weirdness (like waking up from dreams, night terrors, sleep paralysis, sleepwalking or having a hypnic jerk) is normal. We call most unusual things that happen in sleep 'parasomnias'. But when sleep disturbances like this become frequent and disruptive, it's a sign of poor sleep quality or a potential sleep disorder. In my experience in clinic these days, most cases can be improved by working on overall sleep quality and timing of sleep, because in some people, when sleep doesn't serve us, it doesn't just look like taking hours to fall asleep, constant wake-ups or feeling tired but wired and endless thoughts streaming at night instead of sleep – it looks strange. Some of us are just more genetically prone to the weird and wonderful.

This includes me! I've had the occasional night terror – usually when my sleep's been heavily disrupted. One particularly memorable (and not at all fun) episode happened after major knee surgery, when the effects of anaesthesia were still lingering in my system. Anaesthesia can throw off your natural sleep architecture – especially deep sleep – and, in the days after, your brain sometimes rebounds in unpredictable ways. I jumped out of bed mid-terror... straight onto a fully casted leg. Another time, it was stress-related. It was a really intense period in my life, and my brain responded with chaos in the night.

So, if you're constantly exhausted, waking up frequently with night terrors or other parasomnias, or feel unsafe (for example, sleepwalking into things or indeed accidentally hurting your bed partner), it's time to take action. Part 2 will show you how to improve sleep quality naturally. If these methods don't help, it *may* indicate an underlying sleep disorder (covered in the appendix, page 273) which you can also do something about.

Sleep Variation Throughout Our Lives Is Normal

Now you know that sleep is a master of adaptation – it adjusts to sleep debt, redistributes sleep stages when necessary and naturally resists attempts to be hacked. You can't force yourself to get more deep sleep, increase your REM or somehow manipulate your brain to sleep 'better' by targeting one stage. Every stage of sleep, every transition between wakefulness and rest, is controlled by deeply ingrained biological forces. It's a self-regulating system, one that has evolved to help us survive in different environments, from pre-industrial societies to today's artificial-light-filled world. But its adaptability doesn't stop there.

Just as our sleep adjusts in response to these rather large shifts in the way we have lived as humans over time, it can also adapt to the different stages of the human life cycle. What we experience as 'normal sleep' isn't fixed; it evolves as we move through life's 'stuff'.

Sleep is adaptable. It's been adjusting to our environments, our stress levels, our exhaustion levels and our needs since the very beginning – long before we had artificial light, alarm clocks and an obsession with getting eight perfect hours. Sleep has never been a fixed thing, and it never will be.

And yet, somehow, we expect it to be. We assume we should be sleeping the same way in our forties as we did in our twenties. We panic when pregnancy, menopause or ageing changes how we sleep. We worry that if sleep feels different, it must be broken. But here's the truth: sleep changes across our lives because we change across our lives. And the more we learn to work with that instead of against it, the better we'll sleep – not just in terms of how long we sleep, but in how restorative and useful our sleep actually feels.

Sleep isn't meant to be identical every night, and it doesn't need to be perfect to be restorative. Even when sleep feels inconsistent, it can still do its job of helping us recover, repair and function.

Short-term sleep disruptions

There's nothing that sends people into a spiral of sleep anxiety faster than a few bad nights. It's incredible how quickly people go from 'I slept badly last night' to 'What if I never sleep properly again?'

The reality is, short-term sleep disruptions are completely normal. If you're jet-lagged, stressed, recovering from an illness or adjusting to a clock change, of course your sleep is going to feel different. Your entire body is adjusting and, yet, for some reason, we have this expectation that sleep should always stay the same, no matter what's going on. It's ridiculous when you think about it. If we travel across time zones, if we get sick, if we go through stress or major life changes, our whole body reacts – so why wouldn't our sleep be affected too?

People often panic in these situations, thinking that because their sleep feels 'off', they need to immediately do something to fix it. But the best thing you can do for short-term sleep disruptions is absolutely nothing. If you've had a bad night or two, don't start changing your entire routine. Don't start going to bed earlier, waking up later or overthinking every detail of your sleep. Your body is already adapting. The worst thing you can do is interfere with that process.

Take jet lag, for example. People get obsessed with trying to 'force' their sleep into the right time zone, when, actually, their body will do it on its own – if they let it. Instead, they start taking long naps, going to bed at strange times or forcing themselves into an artificial sleep schedule, which just confuses their body further. Or think about stress. If something major is happening in your life, your sleep is probably going to reflect that. You might take longer to fall asleep, wake up more or have more vivid dreams. But that's not sleep failing – that's sleep doing its job. It's adjusting, adapting and working through the mental load you're carrying.

And what about travelling regularly across time zones – say, for work? The mistake many people make is thinking they need to perfectly synchronize to each new location instantly. But your circadian rhythm is not a machine – it doesn't jump to new time zones on command. It shifts gradually, about one to two hours per day, depending on your light exposure. So, if you're a frequent flyer, your body may never fully adjust before you're off again. And that's okay. You don't need to fully adapt to every new time zone. The goal is to reduce unnecessary disruption, not to chase perfect alignment. A strong sleep baseline, as you will learn in this book, helps you tolerate this kind of travel better, even if sleep never feels ideal. (And, by the way, trying harder to fix it usually backfires.)

As for daylight saving time, research shows that even a one-hour shift can temporarily affect sleep and mood, but, again, the key is to *let* your body adjust rather than forcing a fix. One study found that our internal clocks don't shift as fast as the social clock does – and that's where most of the strain comes from. So yes, give yourself a few days to adjust, especially if you're sensitive to changes in morning light. But don't panic. Sleep will recalibrate – just like it always has.

There's also been a lot of media attention around the increase in heart attacks following the spring clock change. And yes, some studies show a small uptick in cardiovascular events right after the shift – likely due to the sudden loss of sleep and circadian misalignment. But the key word here is *small* – we're talking about temporary changes in risk that affect a very specific window of time. If you have a strong sleep baseline and allow time to adjust, the overall impact on your health is minimal. Once again, it's the fear and overcorrection that do more damage than the clock change itself. Besides, heart attack increases happen with other changes, such as the transition between weekends and weekdays – but that doesn't get nearly as much media attention!

The mistake people make is assuming that if their sleep is disrupted, it must mean it's broken. It isn't. In most short-term cases, sleep naturally rights itself once the original trigger passes. The real problem isn't the disruption itself – it's the panic and overcorrection that follows.

So, if you're going through something – whether it's an illness, travel, stress or any other short-term disruptor – your job is to do nothing. Accept that your sleep will be different for a while. Let your body handle it. If things settle on their own, great. If they don't, the following chapters will arm you with some tools and strategies to help deal with them.

But whatever you do, don't start micromanaging your

sleep every time it feels a little off. Because the biggest thing standing between you and better sleep isn't the disruption itself – it's the way you react to it.

'I'm a morning person/night owl'

You've heard it. You've probably said it. But let's pause for a moment – is it entirely true or is it something you've come to believe about yourself? The idea of being a 'night owl' or a 'morning lark' is everywhere now. It's become part of our identities. People wear their late-night energy like a badge of honour: 'Don't talk to me before 10 a.m.!' or 'I get my best ideas at midnight.' While some of us genuinely do have biological tendencies towards later or earlier rhythms (we call these chronotypes and, yes, they are partly genetic), most people have far more control over their sleep timing than they realize.

Chronotypes exist on a spectrum. And while extreme versions – where someone truly can't fall asleep until the early hours and struggles to function before midday – do exist and may warrant further help (we'll talk more about this in the sleep disorder section – see page 273), most of us are not hardwired that way. What we label as our 'chronotype' is often a reflection of our habits, social routines and light-exposure patterns rather than an unchangeable internal truth.

Take one of my former clients, James, a university lecturer who swore he was a classic night owl. He told me his brain only switched on at around 10 p.m. and that, if he could, he'd sleep until 11 a.m. every day. But James had a full-time job and had been waking at 6.30 a.m.

for *years* to get to campus. He never missed a lecture. His body *could* do mornings. He just assumed that the weekend lie-ins and evening energy bursts were proof that he was biologically built for the night shift.

But when we started working on his sleep baseline, which I will also show you how to do, something shifted. Suddenly, his energy started creeping earlier – not forced, not faked, just… naturally. 'I think I've been lying to myself for years,' he told me, half-laughing, half-shocked. 'Turns out I might not be a night owl. I was just inconsistent.'

You might feel groggy in the mornings because you're inconsistent – not because you're a 'bad sleeper' or an owl-for-life. In fact, that grogginess might just be a sign of circadian misalignment, caused by late nights, social jet lag or irregular sleep–wake times – *not a fixed chronotype*.

Chronotype is real, but it's not fixed. It's shaped not only by your genes, but by your light exposure, your habits, your social obligations and your mindset. If you've been telling yourself you're one type for years, maybe it's time to test that theory. What if a few weeks of consistent mornings changed how you feel about evenings?

It's not about becoming a different person – it's about giving your body a fair chance to show you what it can actually do when you stop switching things up all the time. You might still be an evening type, but you might also just be out of sync. The most important thing to understand is that if you're feeling sleep isn't working for you, it's likely we can make it more predictable and stable to serve you better, if this is what you want.

> After all, it's not up to anyone else to tell you what your sleep should be – it just needs to serve you and you alone.

Pregnancy

Pregnancy sleep is a wild ride. I can talk about it from both a professional and very personal perspective, because I'm in the middle of it as I'm writing this. And let me tell you, even when you know exactly what's happening, even when you can explain it scientifically and logically, it still takes you by surprise.

It starts with exhaustion. The kind that makes you want to crawl into bed at 7 p.m. (or, in my case, 11 a.m.!) and sleep for days, except that when you actually do go to bed, sleep feels lighter, more broken and sometimes completely unreachable. It's a cruel joke – your body is demanding more rest while simultaneously making it harder to get. Then there are the vivid dreams, the kind that feel so real and emotionally loaded that you wake up unsure whether they actually happened. I've had some of the most bizarre, intense and occasionally heartbreaking dreams during pregnancy, and I know I'm not alone. This happens because REM sleep shifts during pregnancy, making dream recall more likely. Some nights, it feels like I've lived another entire day in my sleep – sometimes it even feels like therapy, as if my mind is trying to process old material to make room for the new. This doesn't even include all the other seemingly non-related sleep symptoms, such as nausea, stomach cramps and growing pains, but these will also have an impact on our sleep, especially when they occur during sleep time (like so-called 'morning' sickness attacking so many of us at night instead!).

Then, as the months go on, sleep starts breaking apart in a different way. You wake more often, and not just because of bathroom trips or an awkward bump. It's a common experience in pregnancy, particularly in the second and third trimesters, and research confirms that this is when sleep becomes more fragmented. We can't say for certain that this is your body 'practising' for newborn life, but some have speculated that this pattern may be part of how we adapt to what's coming. I love this idea, because even though it's frustrating, it reminds us that sleep might still be looking after us – just not in the way we expect. Personally, I find I'm suddenly more alert if the dog or cat stir (lucky them), and my bladder seems quite pleased with the extra attention too. So I try to take it in my stride, trusting that my body knows what it's doing – even if it's not giving me what I want.

And then there's the discomfort. Finding a comfortable position at night when you're pregnant can feel like a full-time job. You wedge pillows under your bump, between your knees and ankles, behind your back, shifting endlessly to try to create some kind of magic alignment that doesn't leave you aching or numb. It's a delicate balance: one wrong move and suddenly your hip is throbbing, your ribcage feels crushed or your baby has decided that now is the perfect time to do somersaults. You finally settle into a position that feels tolerable, only to realize you need to get up to pee. Again.

There's so much pressure around the 'perfect' pregnancy sleeping position, with advice everywhere telling you to sleep on your left side because it's best for the baby. And while, yes, sleeping on your side, especially the left, is recommended from twenty-eight weeks to support circulation and reduce certain risks, don't panic if you wake up on your back. You're not going to stay in one position all night – your body naturally moves and adjusts. If something feels restrictive, whether for you or your baby, your brain will nudge you awake to shift. That's how sleep works – it protects you without needing constant vigilance. Wonderful!

What's helped me through all of this is expectations. I knew this was coming, so I didn't panic. I didn't lie awake worrying that waking up multiple times meant I was failing at sleep. I didn't tell myself that I needed to 'bank' sleep now before the baby arrives 'because you'll definitely not be getting any then!', as I'm so often told – because you can't bank sleep, that's just not how it works (see Chapter 6 for more on this). I accepted that sleep was going to change, just like everything else in my body, and that's okay. I also feel that perhaps because my sleep baseline/muscle is strong, the effects of pregnancy on my sleep have been more tolerable and less horrid for me. But it also could get worse for me as I make my way through the third trimester... and that's okay too. I am literally building bones in here!

If you want to use this book as a helpful and non-pressured guide to sleep and, most importantly, your mindset around sleep while you go through this ever-changing time, you absolutely can, and should you feel you need further support, please don't hesitate to speak to your medical provider. You are going through a lot and likely your head is buzzing with many things – sleep does not need to be one of them.

Parents and sleep

I spend my life studying sleep, fixing sleep and helping people navigate the overwhelming world of sleep advice. But when it comes to babies and sleep, I am stepping into completely new territory. And, unlike adult sleep – where I have clinical expertise, the scientific background and personal experience – here, I am just a bystander scientist. One thing I know from the adult sleep world is that there is a huge difference between understanding the science of sleep and knowing how to apply that science in real life. There is so much noise out there, so many conflicting opinions and so much pressure to 'get it right' that people are left feeling utterly lost. And from what I've already seen, infant sleep advice is just as chaotic, if not worse, than the advice given to struggling adults.

The messaging is extreme: you're either told you must follow strict routines or that routines are damaging; that sleep training is essential or that sleep training is cruel; that your baby should be sleeping through the night by X months or that night waking is biologically normal forever. And if you're exhausted, struggling and just trying to do the best thing for your child, all this noise doesn't help – it just makes you feel like you're failing, no matter what you do.

So, I'm not going to sit here and fill your head with my ideas on how you should handle your baby's sleep, because I don't believe it's fair for me to do so. If I've learned anything from working in sleep, it's that a scientist with no clinical knowledge – or at the very least, personal experience – should not be advising on how to adapt science to real-world situations. And yet, this is exactly what I see happening in the world of baby (and adult) sleep. That being said, there are a few things I do feel confident about for myself when I navigate this world:

Firstly, every baby is different, and their sleep is supposed to change rapidly at the start. No matter what sleep training method (or lack of method) you use, newborn sleep will evolve quickly and unpredictably. That's how it works. Babies' sleep cycles are shorter, their circadian rhythms are still developing and they are biologically wired to wake frequently. This doesn't mean that sleep guidance isn't useful, but it does mean that rigid expectations can set parents up for a world of frustration.

Secondly, if I find myself struggling, I'm not going to read a thousand different books and Instagram posts until my head explodes. I will do what I always tell my adult clients to do: find one experienced, qualified, evidence-based person/resource to help. I am lucky because I already employ them at Sleepyhead Clinic, but if I didn't, I would still seek out the right professionals or resources.

So, if you're a sleep-deprived parent, my advice isn't about what to do with your baby – it's about what to do with yourself. If you're exhausted and overwhelmed by all the noise, find a source of expertise you trust and stick with it. Don't let the endless cycle of social media, books and well-meaning but contradictory opinions convince you that you're getting it all wrong. You're not. No one knows what they are doing at the beginning and, guess what, all those babies *do* sleep (even if it feels like they *never* sleep) and, eventually, in a way you might be able to cope with!

If there's one thing I do know about sleep – at any age – it's that stress, anxiety and unrealistic expectations will make everything harder. I may not have the answers to infant sleep yet, but I do know this: being kind to yourself in the process is probably the best thing you can do for both you and your baby.

While Part 2 of this book will absolutely help you with your sleep, I want to be realistic about expectations. You won't be able to achieve everything in the same way you might have before having children, because sleep isn't just about you anymore. It's now tied to someone else's needs, rhythms and unpredictability. And that changes things.

But that doesn't mean you can't have good, resilient sleep. It just means that your sleep muscle might look different now – it won't always be about long, uninterrupted nights, but it can still be strong. You can still improve your sleep quality, build up your ability to recover from rough nights and develop a mindset that stops sleep from becoming another source of stress.

Menopause

Menopause is one of those life stages that no one really prepares you for and, when it comes to sleep, it can feel particularly brutal. It's not just a bit of broken sleep here and there – it's full-blown unpredictability. One night you might sleep fine, the next you're awake every hour, soaked in sweat, throwing the duvet off, then shivering and pulling it back on. It's exhausting, frustrating and, just when you think you've adjusted, it changes again. What makes menopause feel so unfair is that it often arrives at a time in life when you finally feel like you should be able to prioritize your own well-being. The kids might be older, and/or your career might be more stable and yet, just as you start thinking, 'Maybe now I'll get some proper rest,' sleep pulls the rug out from under you.

Hormonal shifts – particularly the drop in oestrogen and progesterone – disrupt the way sleep works. They make sleep more fragmented, causing frequent awakenings that feel random, but actually have a lot to do with how hormones interact with sleep regulation. The loss of progesterone, which has a natural calming effect, makes it harder to drift back off after waking, while oestrogen fluctuations wreak havoc on temperature regulation. The result? Hot flushes and night sweats that jolt you awake, only to leave you freezing moments later. It's like your body has decided that regulating temperature is now a full-time job – one that you never applied for.

And it's not just the physical symptoms. Menopause doesn't just affect the body; it affects how you feel about sleep, too. The emotional ups and downs that come with shifting hormones can make broken sleep feel even worse, because it's not just about waking up – it's about waking up angry, frustrated and exhausted in a way that feels deeply personal. The problem is, when sleep starts to feel out of control, the instinct is to try to control it. And this is where a lot of women get stuck. The natural response is to try harder: go to bed earlier, take supplements, follow stricter bedtime routines...

But menopause is a time when the more you try to force sleep, the worse it tends to get. This is because sleep at this stage isn't just about habits – it's about resilience. And resilience isn't built through perfection; it's built through adaptability.

Here's what's interesting: research shows that improving sleep quality before menopause makes menopause easier. Women who have a strong sleep baseline – who have built up a kind of sleep 'muscle' over the years – tend to cope better with the disruption when it comes. This doesn't mean their sleep isn't affected, but it means they can tolerate the changes without spiralling into panic and frustration. They don't chase sleep and, in doing so, they let sleep find its way back to them. I find in clinic that even if they start the process of building a stronger sleep baseline during menopause, there are still significant gains to be had.

The problem is that most of the advice offered for menopausal sleep struggles is about trying to fix it, when what really helps is learning how to navigate it. Menopause isn't something you can outsmart with the perfect routine or by following the endless list of 'sleep hygiene' you may have been presented with when trying to improve sleep, but you can make it significantly more manageable by strengthening your sleep baseline, understanding what's happening and – most importantly – not falling into the trap of thinking that broken sleep means broken health.

We will cover why a lot of the sleep advice out there may not actually work for you in Part 2 (a big hint: because it doesn't really impact your core sleep mechanisms like improving your sleep baseline does). You don't need a 'hack' for menopause sleep; you need a way to get through it without losing your mind. And, trust me, that's absolutely possible.

How sleep changes as we age

As we get older, our sleep naturally changes, and one of the biggest shifts is that we get less deep sleep. This isn't something to worry about – it's a normal part of how our brain reorganizes itself with age. As we've seen, deep sleep, or stage 3 sleep, is when the body focuses on physical repair, muscle growth, immune function and clearing waste from the brain. When we're young, we need a lot of it because our bodies and brains are still developing. But as we age, we don't need as much deep sleep for these processes, and so our sleep cycles adjust.

This shift happens for a few reasons. The brain itself changes over time, and some of the neurons responsible for generating deep sleep activity gradually become less active. There's also a hormonal link – the production of growth hormone, which is closely tied to deep sleep, naturally declines as we get older, so the body spends less time in deep sleep simply because it doesn't need as much of it. Our circadian rhythm also shifts, making us naturally more inclined to fall asleep and wake up earlier. On top of that, sleep cycles become a little more fragmented, which can make sleep feel lighter or more interrupted, even though it's still doing its job. Very light stages like REM get even easier to wake up from, given all the new interruptions like pain, bladder breaks or the side effects of medications.

The key thing to understand is that having less deep sleep doesn't necessarily mean our sleep is worse. The body compensates in other ways, and it continues to adapt. Lighter sleep stages, which increase with age, are still beneficial for things like memory processing and regulating emotions. And while deep sleep is restorative, it's not the only part of sleep that matters. The brain adjusts how it uses sleep based on what it needs, and as long as sleep feels generally refreshing, a drop in deep sleep isn't something to panic about.

That being said, some older adults do feel that their sleep isn't as good as it used to be. This isn't always because of changes in deep sleep itself, but rather how those changes are perceived. Many people assume that because sleep feels different, it must be broken, which can create stress and anxiety that actually disrupts sleep further. Other factors can also play a role, like chronic pain, medication side effects or spending less time outside, which affects circadian rhythm regulation.

The mistake people often make is trying to force sleep to look like it did in their twenties, when, in reality, the goal should be to work with these natural changes rather than against them. Instead of obsessing over getting more deep sleep, the focus should be on maintaining overall sleep quality – making sure that sleep, even if it's lighter or more broken, still feels restorative. And if it doesn't, I would argue, just like at any age, it is not due to the original trigger like ageing, but the beliefs and behaviours that came after. That's when we can absolutely improve sleep to a new baseline that serves you right now.

Sleep isn't meant to stay the same throughout our lives, and the fact that it evolves is a sign that it's still doing exactly what it's supposed to do: adjusting to meet our needs. The more we learn to trust it, rather than fight it, the better we'll sleep.

Does this mean we need to tolerate chronic poor sleep that really is affecting our quality of life? No, not at all, even if we know what's triggering it and it seems insurmountable. Part 2 will address how you can keep your sleep muscle strong and have a good sleep baseline, making all of this life change and sleep variation much less significant and far more tolerable.

Neurodiversity and Sleep: When Your Brain Plays by Its Own Rules

Some people spend their whole lives feeling like sleep is just a little... off. Not broken, necessarily, but different

– harder to settle into, harder to maintain and never quite as refreshing as it seems to be for everyone else. For a lot of people, this isn't just random bad luck, it's because their brain works differently, so their sleep does too.

Take attention deficit hyperactivity disorder (ADHD). A lot of people with ADHD struggle with sleep in a way that doesn't make sense on paper. They can be utterly exhausted but wired, unable to shut their brain down at night. Then, when they do finally sleep, they wake up feeling just as tired as when they went to bed. It's not that they don't get enough sleep (although that's often the case too); it's that the transitions between sleep stages don't happen as smoothly. Their circadian rhythm is often naturally delayed, so they feel tired later than they 'should'. Their brains don't downshift into sleep as efficiently, and some research suggests they might spend less time in deep sleep and more time in lighter, less restorative sleep. The end result? Sleep feels unreliable, even when they technically get enough of it.

Autism presents its own set of challenges when it comes to sleep. Many autistic people have sensory sensitivities that can make sleep feel fragile. A slightly scratchy bedsheet, a change in room temperature or even a minor shift in bedtime routine can be enough to disrupt sleep in a way that feels disproportionate. Some research also suggests that autistic people produce melatonin differently, which may be why many struggle with falling asleep at a 'normal' time. It's not that sleep is impossible, but it often requires a level of consistency that the rest of the world doesn't always allow for.

And then there are conditions like bipolar disorder, where sleep feels like it's either too much or too little, depending on where someone is in their cycle. Or chronic fatigue syndrome (CFS), where sleep feels utterly unrefreshing, no matter how much of it you get. Or anxiety and depression, which tend to increase REM sleep but also fragment it, leaving people waking up feeling more emotionally drained than when they went to bed.

For all of these conditions, the biggest mistake people make is assuming that if their sleep isn't 'normal', it must be broken. But sleep in these cases isn't necessarily failing – it's just playing by a different set of rules. Trying to force it into a neurotypical or 'one-size-fits-all' model is where the frustration comes in.

Instead of chasing perfect sleep, the real goal should be about understanding how your own sleep naturally works and figuring out how to support it, rather than fighting against it. That doesn't mean settling for terrible sleep – it just means approaching it from a place of adjustment, not force.

Chronic Illness and Sleep: When Rest Feels Unrefreshing

Chronic illness changes everything – your energy, your body and your ability to function day to day. So, of course, it changes sleep too. And yet, this is one of the hardest things for people to accept. There's often this expectation that no matter what's going on in the body, sleep should still 'fix' things.

Pain conditions like arthritis, fibromyalgia and other chronic pain disorders make sleep feel light, broken and frustrating. Pain wakes you up. Finding a comfortable position takes work. And even when you do sleep, it can feel like it hasn't done what it's supposed to do – because you still wake up exhausted.

People with conditions like myalgic encephalomyelitis (ME)/CFS often describe sleep as feeling like it's 'not working' at all. They can sleep ten, twelve hours and still feel completely wiped out, as if sleep just isn't restoring them the way it should. Research backs this up: there's evidence that the way the brain cycles through sleep in these conditions may be altered, meaning restorative sleep doesn't happen as efficiently.

The hardest part of all of this? Expectations. People assume that if they sleep long enough, they should feel better. But chronic illness changes the equation. The body is working harder than usual and, sometimes, even good sleep can't undo that.

So what's the answer? The same as always: not chasing perfection, but figuring out what works for you. That might mean adjusting routines, changing expectations or focusing more on how to improve daily energy rather than seeing sleep as the ultimate fix-all. It's not about giving up on sleep. It's about understanding that when the body is under strain, sleep is just one piece of a much bigger puzzle.

Everything you have learned so far is how sleep works, how aligned it is with our environment and planet, and how it adapts over time, but this contrasts wildly with our current sleep culture. How did we get to this contradiction? We will explore this further in the next chapter.

CHAPTER 2

How We Got So Weird About Sleep – and Why It's Making Us Sleep Worse

Imagine trying to explain to your medieval great-great-great-grandmother that you spent £300 on a watch that tells you whether you slept well. She'd probably laugh in your face and say, 'Did you wake up alive? Great, sounds like a good night's sleep to me.' Yet, here we are, obsessing over sleep scores and panicking if we didn't get our eight hours. So, how did we get here? How did we go from sleep being something you just do, to being something you try to win at? How did we go from sleep being something natural to something we obsess over? First, we treated it like a mystery. Then, we treated it like an obstacle. Finally, we treated it like a performance – and that's when things went seriously wrong.

For most of history, sleep was boring. It just happened. When humans first started to contemplate what sleep was, it was generally accepted that it was a natural part of life, passive and mysterious. It just wasn't obvious what sleep was; therefore, the simplest explanation was usually taken: a shutdown mode for the body, barely worth studying.

Even when philosophers and early doctors thought about sleep, it was usually a side note to bigger questions. There were more pressing matters – like staying alive through plagues. Sleep wasn't seen as something to master; it was just a fact of life.

Some cultures understood sleep as having religious or spiritual significance; for example, the Egyptians thought our dreams were messages from the gods, but nobody was lying awake thinking, 'Did I get enough REM?'

Then came the Industrial Revolution. Suddenly, as we saw in Chapter 1, sleep got in the way of progress. You couldn't be a good factory worker if you were snoozing. Shift work, clocks and artificial light turned sleep into a problem – something that interfered with productivity: 'I'll sleep when I'm dead.' And, indeed, they probably got there faster.

The Science Breakthrough – and the Anxiety It Sparked

Fast-forward to the twentieth century, when science started peeking under the hood of sleep. First, we discovered that the brain wasn't just shutting off – it was busy! The electroencephalogram (EEG) showed sleep was an active process. Then REM sleep was discovered, showing that sleep is anything but passive. We started realizing that sleep is vital for memory, learning, immunity... you name it. But here's where it went wrong: once we realized sleep was critical to health – and that not getting enough could hurt us – it made sense to want more of it. But rather than asking how sleep works best, we fixated on one thing: how long.

Focusing on the wrong things

Here's the frustrating part about this: we actually do know what makes sleep work now. Science has given us two incredible insights: your circadian rhythm and sleep drive (which we looked at in Chapter 1). These are the real engines of sleep. The big players. The behind-the-scenes heroes that run the whole show. And we've known about them for decades.

Circadian rhythms were first hinted at way back in the eighteenth century, when scientists noticed that plants still followed light–dark cycles even when kept in constant darkness – as if they had an internal clock ticking away. But it wasn't until the 1950s and 60s, through human isolation experiments (where people lived in caves for weeks), that we confirmed humans have their own built-in clock, too.

Sleep drive came onto the scene a little later, when researchers started to understand homeostasis – the process by which your body maintains balance. In the 1970s and 80s, scientists realized that, just as we build hunger the longer we go without food, we also build up a biological pressure to sleep the longer we're awake.

But what did we do with this knowledge? We got distracted. We threw out the user manual and fixated on one tiny, misleading metric. Instead of asking, 'How do I work with my body clock and sleep drive to get good-quality sleep?' we ask, 'Did I get eight hours?' as if that number alone holds some magic power.

But here's the truth: it doesn't. By focusing only on how long we sleep, we've missed the bigger picture – and, in doing so, we've made sleep harder. We've forgotten that sleep is a dynamic process that responds to what we do during the day, how much light we get and how consistent our rhythms are. Instead, we lie in bed, watching the clock, stressing that we're not 'hitting the target'.

It's like owning a car, knowing full well it runs on both petrol and a battery, but only ever checking how much petrol is in the tank. Meanwhile, the battery's flat, and you're wondering why the engine won't start.

Sleep duration is not the whole story; it's not necessarily the most important part. Yet, it's the thing that dominates every conversation we have about sleep, every headline, every app. As a result, people don't know about circadian rhythm and sleep drive – the very systems that would actually help them sleep better.

So, while it's amazing that we've discovered so much about how sleep works, we've also done something incredibly human: we've taken something complex and boiled it down to a number and, in doing so, we've made the whole situation worse.

How did this happen?

Over the last decade, sleep has been elevated to an almost sacred status – and rightly so. Thanks to bestselling books like *Why We Sleep* and *The Sleep Revolution*, and a growing body of accessible science, sleep has finally been recognized as fundamental to health. This is a welcome shift after decades of it being sidelined or misunderstood.

But with this new spotlight has also come a shadow. As a clinician, I've started to notice a rising tide of sleep anxiety – not just in my patients, but in everyday conversations with friends and across the media. The message that sleep is important has sometimes been translated into a rigid belief that it must also be perfect – or else.

'You'd be so disappointed in me,' a friend said recently, half-joking, but clearly a bit worried. 'I didn't go to bed early and I forgot to have a warm bath!' These aren't unusual comments – and they reflect something deeper. Somewhere along the way, the well-meaning guidance about sleep has become a checklist for moral success. And when people feel they've failed at sleep, it doesn't just affect their night, it affects how they feel about themselves the next day.

On top of that, the advice itself in my friend's example is just wrong. It's not the most important thing you can do to improve your sleep and, for many people, it may make no difference at all – in fact, it could even make things worse if you start over-focusing on doing everything 'perfectly'.

The Problem with the Sleep Deprivation Narrative

One of the most harmful stories we tell ourselves today is that we're all walking around chronically sleep-deprived; that any time sleep looks different – shorter, broken, lighter – we must be damaging ourselves. But when you really look at the evidence, this isn't true. Not only are most people's sleep systems far more resilient than this narrative suggests, but the studies that support these sweeping claims are often misinterpreted, poorly designed or presented out of context.

One of the most worrying stories we tell ourselves today is that we're all walking around chronically sleep-deprived.

Not everyone is sleep-deprived just because sleep looks different

Let's be clear: chronic sleep deprivation – the kind that truly threatens health – is actually difficult to achieve without it rapidly becoming obvious and dangerous. This is not just theoretical: the human body cannot sustain sleep deprivation without profound mental and physical collapse. Have you ever tried to keep yourself awake for long periods of time? It's actually really hard to do! If chronic, severe sleep deprivation were something people could quietly endure for years, it wouldn't be an effective form of torture – but it is, and always has been.

Yet, the way sleep deprivation is discussed in public health messaging today would have us believe that most people are walking around on the edge of collapse – just because their sleep doesn't hit eight hours every night. That simply doesn't hold up when you look closely at the data – or clinic, where people are not dropping down dead from lack of sleep.

Here's the problem: most studies that drive this fear narrative about sleep deprivation fail to properly distinguish between sleep duration and sleep quality. They group together people who sleep short amounts but have good sleep with those who sleep short amounts and have fragmented, poor-quality sleep – and then they attribute the health outcomes to sleep duration alone, rather than recognizing that it's usually poor quality or disrupted sleep that could be driving the risk.

This point is critical. The Penn State cohort studies on sleep and mortality found that significantly higher mortality risk was associated with people who had both **short sleep duration and poor-quality, unrefreshing sleep**, not those who simply slept fewer hours. Yet, this nuance rarely makes it into the public conversation. Instead, we hear the simplified message: 'short sleep kills'. But that's not what the research showed. People who naturally sleep fewer hours and feel well-rested – so-called 'short, good-quality sleepers' – did *not* show those same mortality risks.

Other large-scale reviews support this. An umbrella review in *Frontiers in Medicine* found that poor sleep quality amplifies the health risks of short sleep – not short sleep alone. And critically, another meta-analysis found that long sleep durations – often assumed to be healthier – were also linked to increased mortality, particularly when sleep was fragmented or associated with underlying health problems. So, both short and long sleep are linked to risks when quality is poor, not because of the number of hours alone.

These nuances matter. Because what's driving many people's fear is the idea that sleep must be long, perfect and unbroken to be healthy, which is not what the science says. The data we rely on to make these sweeping claims about sleep are often based on flawed measurements.

Another problem rarely discussed is how sleep is measured in many of these studies. Much of the research is based on self-reported sleep data, which is known to be inaccurate. People are terrible at estimating how much they actually sleep, especially if they experience light sleep or normal night-time awakenings (which they mistake for being awake).

In fact, polysomnography (gold standard sleep studies) consistently shows that people with insomnia, for example, often sleep much more than they think they do – but because they are aware of light sleep, they perceive that they haven't slept at all during this stage. So when studies report 'short sleepers', we have to ask: are these true short sleepers or just people who perceive their sleep to be short? And if it's perception, is it the short sleep that causes health issues or the anxiety, stress and hyperarousal that comes from thinking you're sleep-deprived?

This distinction matters because our perception of sleep – especially when shaped by fear and expectation – can drive physiological stress responses, which may explain some of the observed health risks rather than just number of hours slept.

There is no single 'right' duration of sleep – and chasing it can do more harm than good. For years, we've been told we need eight hours of sleep. More recently, there's been a shift to seven hours as a new magic number, and it's likely to change again. But here's the truth: there is no universal sleep duration that applies to everyone (even if there were, you wouldn't be able to get it every night, and you can't make it happen just by knowing).

Large-scale genetic and population studies show huge individual variability in sleep need. Yes, there are outliers and they are rare – natural very short sleepers and very long sleepers – but also a wide, normal range in between. As we saw in the last chapter, people's needs change across their lifespan, with age, health status, genetics and environment playing a role. To insist that everyone needs the same duration is as nonsensical as saying everyone should eat the same number of calories, regardless of size, age or activity level.

Here's why this matters: forcing people to chase a specific number of hours can drive anxiety and worsen sleep. It leads people to spend longer in bed, overextending their sleep window, which we know fragments sleep and leads to lighter, more broken sleep – the very thing that causes health risks in the first place. So, in trying to hit an arbitrary target, we're causing the very problems we fear.

Even when both short duration and poor quality exist, these outcomes are not fixed – sleep is adaptable and can improve.

Finally, even when people do show both short sleep and poor sleep quality – the combination linked with higher mortality – these outcomes are not set in stone. Improving sleep quality can significantly reduce risk, even if total sleep time doesn't increase.

In fact, focusing on building a strong, consistent sleep rhythm and working with circadian alignment and sleep drive (rather than chasing more hours) can restore functional, restorative sleep – and that is what improves health outcomes. Yet, this hopeful and practical message is rarely emphasized in public discussions about sleep, which remain fixated on duration.

These are the key things I wish were common knowledge and, perhaps together, we can make them so:

1. Chronic, true sleep deprivation is difficult to achieve without rapid, obvious collapse and, most importantly, falling asleep at any opportunity – and isn't the everyday reality for most people.
2. Most people who think they're sleep-deprived are not necessarily – they're victims of flawed studies and fear-driven narratives.
3. Studies driving the fear focus on duration, but often fail to separate it from quality, and they depend on unreliable self-reporting.
4. There is no universal sleep need – and forcing a duration causes more problems than it solves.
5. Even in high-risk groups, sleep quality improvement can reduce risk – sleep is adaptable, not broken forever.

Culture made sleep a performance

Now, imagine someone who underestimates their sleep and then believes poor sleep quality means any break in sleep – can you see how the anxiety and stress that this must cause alone is going to have an impact on sleep itself?

Technology has only added fuel to the fire. You might think tracking more sleep metrics would help, but when the goal is perfection, not understanding, they just reinforce the same old myths.

Sleep trackers, apps and gadgets have turned rest into something to be measured, scored and perfected. People wake up to numbers that tell them whether their sleep was good or bad, often feeling worse when their data doesn't match their expectations, even if they feel fine. Indeed, in the research, we see that even when a tracker deliberately lies about your sleep data being bad, it will drive poor health outcomes during the day. While intended to be something useful, devices like this, when not designed well, can mislead us into thinking that we can micromanage sleep.

And then there are social media, where influencers peddle misinformation and trends like mouth-taping, sleep supplements and even 'bed-rotting' (spending extra time in bed as a form of self-care). These trends don't tend to fix anything, because they don't consider those core sleep mechanisms: the circadian rhythm and sleep drive. Yet, they are popular because of the confusion, fear and lack of good resources in sleep medicine.

This cultural fixation has also contributed to a rise in sleep perfectionism – the relentless drive to 'perform' sleeping well. A good example of this is the increase in 'orthosomnia' (*ortho* meaning straight or correct, and *somnia* meaning sleep – coined by research teams looking at the effects of things like sleep tracking), a modern sleep disorder in which people develop insomnia because they're so anxious about achieving perfect sleep.

While well-meaning, sleep hygiene trends, routines and rituals have often done more harm than good. For many people, these practices lead to shame and guilt when sleep doesn't go to plan. If you are continually told that simply relaxing before bed, for example, will fix your sleep issues, you're made to feel that there's something wrong with you if it doesn't work. The mindset isolates us, makes us feel lonely and makes us feel that something is awry with our internal sleep systems (even though most advice and tips don't consider the sleep system!). This, in turn, makes sleep problems harder to fix even with the right advice, as you lose faith in your own ability and don't want to trust anything else.

It doesn't help that sleep science, while growing, remains a relatively young and underfunded field because of how long it took us to understand. There aren't enough qualified sleep experts and reliable sleep resources to guide people through these challenges, and the vacuum has been filled by influencers, oversimplified advice and a commercial market pushing supplements and gadgets. And while technology has dramatically advanced very quickly, our thinking has not, so we are not yet equipped to understand or deal with all the extra data in a way that helps rather than hinders us.

This isn't just a funny cultural shift – it's actually making sleep worse. The more people worry, the more they interfere with the natural process of sleep. It's like trying to force yourself to fall asleep, which we all know is impossible. The pursuit of perfect sleep has become the very thing that ruins it.

Like many clinical sleep physiologists and sleep doctors, I have watched my clinics go from genuine cases of chronic sleep disorders to general anxiety about sleep. I've even had people in clinic resort to lying about how little sleep they've had, because they think that's the only way to convince a professional that they need help. This anxiety, when not dealt with quickly, can turn into a very real and severe sleep disorder, insomnia. We can avoid this.

Let's get practical. We've just pulled apart the mess, how we used to treat sleep as something boring and automatic, and how we've somehow turned it into a competitive sport full of rules, fear and overthinking. We've looked at how we lost sight of the basics, and how the culture around sleep has started doing more harm than good. From this point on, we'll get stuck into the practical stuff – not a list of tips or tricks, but real, useful ways to get your sleep back on track, based on how it actually works.

If you've ever thought, 'Why can everyone else sleep through chaos and I'm wide awake because of a tap dripping?', then you're going to want to keep reading. Let's talk about what's really going on – and how to get your sleep system feeling a bit more solid again.

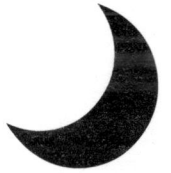

PART 2

SLEEP 2.0: YOUR NEW SLEEP OPERATING SYSTEM

CHAPTER 3

Sleep Sensitivity: The Dripping Tap, the Ticking Clock...

The problem: As people become hypersensitive to sleep triggers (for example, stress or changes in routine), their sleep gets worse and they wake up more at night, leading to a vicious cycle.

The fix: Reverse-engineering: instead of getting distracted by the trigger, focus more holistically on your sleep. Treat sleep as the condition, not the symptom of another. Keep the 'sleep muscle' strong, and you will notice less broken sleep.

We now know that sleep variation can be normal. Learning to accept this can prevent interference, which in turn can lead to more stable sleep (even though, remember, sleep cannot be perfect all the time). But, let's be honest, when it's 3 a.m. and the dog's snoring sounds like a freight train or the streetlight is practically giving your bedroom an X-ray, all that rational thinking goes out the window... We're starting Part 2 with one of the most common things we likely all go through at some point or another – something that sneaks up on people without them realizing: sleep sensitivity.

The Overly Sensitive Sleeper

Have you ever wondered how your bed partner is sleeping soundly through the loudest, most insistent ticking clock, restless pet or dripping tap while you feel like you're lying in the middle of a construction site? It's not uncommon to suddenly become hypersensitive to the world around you when you're trying to sleep. And no, you're not imagining it. The phenomenon is real. You're not 'weaker' or 'wired wrong'. What's actually happening is that your brain has started overreacting to stimuli because it's been trained by broken sleep.

This hypersensitivity doesn't happen overnight (pun fully intended). It's part of a vicious cycle. The more a trigger breaks your sleep – whether it's an overactive bladder, noisy neighbours or stress from an ongoing work problem – the more your sleep becomes broken. The more broken your sleep gets, the more sensitive you become to that original trigger and other, more benign ones. Before long, you start calling yourself a 'light sleeper' and resign yourself to a life of disrupted nights.

But let me tell you: no one is born a 'light sleeper'. It's not a genetic condition passed down from your mother's side of the family. Instead, it's a behaviour your brain learns over time – an unhelpful adaptation to broken sleep. And the very fact your brain can learn unhelpful habits is a sign that it can also unlearn them.

Why fixing the trigger rarely fixes the problem

Most people assume the original trigger is the culprit behind their new-found sensitivity and focus all their energy on fixing it. Logical, right? Well, yes and no.

Take stress as an example. I've had clients who became utterly consumed with eliminating their stress to improve their sleep, diving headfirst into mindfulness apps, relaxation techniques and every 'mind-clearing' strategy under the sun. And while these things are helpful in isolation, they didn't fix their sleep. Why? Because the original trigger wasn't the whole story – not anymore. By the time they came to me, their sleep sensitivity had taken on a life of its own.

Let's break this down: if you can truly eradicate a trigger in its earliest stages – say, within the first few days or weeks – and you already have a strong sleep baseline, you might avoid this hypersensitivity altogether. But once the cycle sets in, it's no longer just about the trigger.

Your brain has learned to associate wakefulness with that trigger.

Fixating on one trigger to fix your sleep once that hypersensitivity has kicked in is like trying to stop a leaky pipe by just wiping up the puddle – over and over *and over* again. Sure, you're managing the symptoms, but the problem isn't going anywhere until you address the bigger picture.

How the Brain Makes You a Light Sleeper

One of the most common triggers for sleep sensitivity is noise. At night, your brain's reticular activating system (RAS) helps filter out sounds so you can stay asleep. But when your sleep is repeatedly disturbed, this system goes into overdrive, making you hyper-aware of every creak, cough and cat meow. Chronic broken sleep doesn't just mess with your RAS, it can also hijack your amygdala – the part of your brain that processes fear and threat – putting it on high alert. Now, even harmless sounds feel intrusive, and the cycle deepens. Broken sleep can increase stress hormones like cortisol, making your brain even more alert at night and not ready to sleep.

This is why your partner, who snores like a congested walrus, can blissfully sleep through your angry pokes while you lie awake fuming. Their brain hasn't assigned 'danger' to those noises. Your brain, however, is staging a full-blown intervention at the slightest rustle of the duvet.

Here's where it gets even more frustrating. Your brain is incredibly adaptable, which is a double-edged sword. It 'learns' to wake up to these harmless triggers because it thinks it's helping you. The more this happens, the more your brain rewires itself to function on broken sleep.

There's robust research to support this. Studies on chronic insomniacs have found that even after years of sleep disruption, their brains develop compensatory mechanisms to perform cognitively on par with non-insomniacs in tasks like attention and memory. While this adaptability is fascinating, it reinforces how deeply ingrained these patterns become – and why breaking them requires focused intervention.

I've had clients who, against all odds, managed to eliminate their original triggers. One woman finally sorted out her overactive bladder with medical treatment, only to find herself still waking up every fifty-five minutes. She was dumbfounded. 'But I fixed it!' she said. The truth? It was too late – her brain had already hardwired the broken sleep pattern.

When rational thinking goes out the window

We've all been there, lying in bed at night, spiralling into irrational thoughts about why we're awake: 'I'll never sleep again!', 'I'm going to be a complete disaster at work tomorrow!' or, my favourite, 'This one bad night means I'm going to die ten years earlier!' The irony is, these thoughts are fuelled by the same brain that's trying to keep you awake. It's your fight-or-flight system, working overtime to 'protect' you from sleep triggers. In reality, these thoughts only perpetuate the cycle of stress and sleeplessness. We will discuss sleep anxiety in more detail in Chapter 5, because your brain has to get these thoughts from somewhere, and they are very powerful even without sensitivity. We are not nocturnal creatures, and therefore your brain doesn't work the same way as it does during the day – this is why we are prone to such irrational, even paranoid thinking in the middle of the night. So, give yourself a break: yes, you have suddenly become completely irrational, but so has everyone else.

Why society makes it worse

Let's take a moment to talk about how lonely sleep problems can feel. Everyone else seems to brag about how they 'hit the pillow and they're gone', as if this is some gold standard of human functionality. Meanwhile, you're lying there wondering why your brain won't shut up about whether the curtains are fully closed.

And then there's the endless parade of well-meaning but useless advice: 'Just come off your phone,' they say. 'Relax before bed, and you'll be fine!' Oh, really? So how do you explain the people scrolling TikTok for hours and still sleeping like logs? This mismatch between advice and reality only deepens the sense of frustration and isolation.

The Worst Mistake in Treating Sleep Problems

The worst thing we ever do when encountering sleep problems is seeing them as a symptom of something else, instead of treating the sleep issue as the primary concern. Qualified medical professionals are often, ironically, the worst at doing this, and it leads us down all sorts of mostly unhelpful paths when it comes to sleep. While sleep problems often start with an initial trigger like illness, new medication, environmental changes, too much time on your phone before bed, stress... you name it, by the time most people seek out support for sleep, the sleep problem has been learned. It's a new sleep pattern that isn't simply going to go away just because you solve all your problems.

This is a story I get told a lot:

> I did go to the doctors because I became desperate and, at first, they fobbed me off with basic sleep hygiene and to de-stress, which I had already done before I went to the doctor. Then they told me I had depression and prescribed antidepressants! I left feeling like I hadn't been listened to and that there

must be something really wrong with me – I must be different from everyone else.

Now, no shade on doctors, who are feeling much the same as the public when it comes to sleep – most wish there was more education on sleep so they didn't feel underprepared and pressured when diagnosing and managing sleep issues, which, unfortunately, often leads to misdiagnosis or inappropriate treatments. Surveys of educational providers show that sleep medicine is one of the most under-taught areas during medical training, with many doctors receiving fewer than two hours of sleep-related education.

When your doctor hands you a leaflet that says, 'Have you tried avoiding caffeine before bed?', it's like being told to check if the TV is plugged in when it won't turn on. (And while reducing coffee can help if you notice that your sleep problem started when you went from two to fifteen cups a day, it will not do a thing to resolve your particular issue if this was not the case.)

Why this needs to change

We have to change how we deal with sleep problems because not only are these approaches not fixing the issues, or indeed making them worse, but there is another side effect: not being acknowledged in the right way, and fobbing people off with the wrong answer, makes us feel unheard, lonely and isolated. This in itself is a big problem. Sleep problems can already feel alienating – the hours spent wide awake in the dark, believing you're the only one in the world awake – but this isolation is compounded when no one seems to understand what you're going through, not even your doctor.

And when someone feels ignored or dismissed, it erodes their confidence in finding a solution. By the time they reach me, they've often lost faith in themselves, in the idea that sleep can get better or even in proper scientific medical care. This creates an uphill battle, as faith in the process is crucial for sleep recovery. Without confidence, it's like trying to learn to swim while clinging to the side of the pool – you're too afraid to let go and trust the process.

Reverse-Engineering Sleep

Based on hundreds of clients I've worked with (and much research!), the solution lies in what I like to call 'reverse-engineering sleep': start with the sleep, not the trigger. Sleep isn't just a symptom of something else – it's a condition in itself. Treat it like a muscle that needs strengthening. When you do this, triggers lose their power over you.

If you train for a marathon by only running when you feel like it, you're not going to get very far. Sleep is no different.

Strengthening your sleep baseline

Think of it this way: if you train for a marathon by only running when you feel like it, you're not going to get very far. Sleep is no different. A strong baseline isn't about perfection – it's about consistency in the most influential simple things over time.

Imagine your sleep like a house foundation. If the foundation's weak, the whole structure above becomes unstable. Building a strong sleep baseline is like reinforcing that foundation, so, when life inevitably throws storms your way (illness, a newborn, a big work project), your house might sway a little, but it won't collapse.

The key to calming sleep sensitivity is consistency over time. Keep the sleep muscle strong – not just when things go wrong, but every day, in small, manageable ways. It's not about doing everything right or living like a monk. It's about understanding how your sleep works, so it can start working *for* you again.

And that's where we're headed next. Let's walk through the key things you can do to *build* that foundation.

CHAPTER 4

Why Your Morning Matters More Than Your Evening

The problem: The obsession with evening routines, bedtime, catching up and the lie-in paradox.

The fix: Your morning habits, especially consistent wake times and light exposure, are far more impactful than any evening routine. I'll show you how timing and light anchor your circadian rhythms.

What if everything you thought you knew about fixing your sleep was backwards? For years, we've been bombarded with advice about the perfect evening routine: lavender sprays, meditation apps, bedtime yoga, no screens for two hours before bed... The commercial sleep industry has turned nighttime into a ritualistic battleground, where your ability to relax 'just right' is supposedly the key to better sleep.

But what if I told you that none of this matters as much as what you do in the morning?

In this chapter, I'm going to take everything we've covered so far and help you put it into action. This isn't about striving for perfection or adding more pressure to your bedtime. It's about helping you reset your sleep by starting at the right end of the day: your morning. We'll walk through the simple but powerful things you can start doing the moment you wake up – things that can dramatically improve your sleep quality, energy levels and resilience. We've talked about building a strong sleep baseline, and this is how you achieve it. Whether you're dealing with full-blown insomnia or just stuck in a cycle of groggy mornings and unpredictable nights, this is where things can really start to shift.

That's right: the secret to better sleep doesn't start with your evening – it starts with your morning habits. Forget about evening wind-down routines, early bedtimes or the idea of 'catching up' on sleep with a luxurious weekend lie-in. These well-meaning strategies might feel like you're doing something productive, but often they're traps that disrupt your natural sleep–wake cycle, leaving you groggy and stuck in a frustrating loop.

Let's be honest: how many times have you tried to get yourself to sleep earlier, only to lie awake staring at the ceiling? How often have you enjoyed a glorious weekend lie-in, only to feel even more tired on Monday morning? Or doubled down on evening relaxation rituals, expecting miracles, and woken up just as exhausted?

Your morning habits – especially your wake-up time, light exposure and movement – are more powerful in determining how well you sleep than anything you do in the evening. Your circadian rhythm is far more obsessed with consistency than relaxation. It cares about when you get up, how much light you see and whether your body gets the signals it needs to wake up and stay awake.

I'm going to show you why mornings matter so much and give you practical, science-backed ways to reset your sleep from the moment you open your eyes. By the end of this chapter, you'll understand why 'catching up' on sleep and rigid evening routines often backfire – and how building better mornings can make sleep effortless again.

Going to Bed Early: Why It Doesn't Work

Most people will take to their beds when they feel sleep needs to be resolved. Let's take a recent client of mine, Suli. Suli owns a small but very popular Turkish café with her brother. A single mum, she has two teenage children, two dogs and a beautiful new build she worked hard to create, now twenty years into their business. Suli is postmenopausal and on HRT, which she feels has given her 'mental balance' but has not been particularly useful for physical symptoms, like sleep. Suli's days can be long and hard – she runs the kitchen of the café, but is also managing the entire business, even on her days off. Suli's sleep in the last few years has become very broken and unfulfilling, alongside the exhaustion she already feels from such an active twenty-four-hour job. Naturally, when work has been long and she has looked after her family and walked the dogs, going to bed early feels like the right thing to do.

So, why isn't simply adding more sleep opportunity helping here? It's a myth that more time in bed always leads to better sleep quality. Studies show that spending too much time in bed can actually lead to 'sleep fragmentation' – short, interrupted sleep cycles that leave us feeling unrefreshed.

This is a common story I hear when a client with insomnia describes how their sleep problem started and what they did to try to resolve it, only to find it getting worse – and now it's chronic, debilitating insomnia that seems unshifting and immoveable. I appreciate that a lot of you reading this aren't in Suli's position yet, with a chronic sleep problem, but this is often partly how insomnia starts for a lot of people, and I want you to avoid this.

Can't you 'catch up'?

Sometimes, if you're already a good sleeper and lose a few hours due to an unexpected event, you can 'catch up' by going to bed early the following night. But for those who struggle with regular sleep inconsistency, relying on extra hours often backfires, creating further disruption. That's because your body's sleep needs aren't just about clocking hours but about maintaining consistent wake and sleep patterns over time. Our internal clock, or circadian rhythm, relies on consistency; it's set up to expect predictable sleep patterns. Each time we vary our sleep timing – whether it's by catching up or staying up – the brain's internal 'sleep drive' gets confused, making it harder to fall and stay asleep.

And 'willing' sleep to come, unfortunately, doesn't make it so. When sleep becomes forced, the brain shifts out of 'rest mode' and into a heightened state that actually blocks sleep.

When we sleep can have just as much impact as how much we sleep.

The lie-in paradox

I am convinced, after twenty years of exploring the sleep world, that lying in has been built on a commercial conspiracy. Why are we obsessed with lie-ins?! Ask yourself, why do we think that the 7 a.m. energized runner is 'wild', but lying in a dark room at the weekend during your free time when you don't have to work is normal? I mean, think about it – you finally have some free time, but you just want to lie there in the dark and,

When we sleep can have just as much impact as how much we sleep.

when you do force yourself to get up, it's for work! I'll admit I was exactly the same, indoctrinated into this 'lying in is a luxury' idea, until I went to work at Harvard Sleep Labs on some very interesting circadian studies that blew my tiny little mind.

When I picture lying in, I think of bed adverts and cosying up with a cup of tea (preferably brought to me) with the animals (including the husband) on soft luxury bedding on a super comfy bed. I think this vision of luxury is powerful. It's often marketed as the ultimate form of relaxation. Companies sell the idea that a lie-in is self-care, ignoring any real science on our sleep-and-wake health. What they don't show is the reality of things. They rarely mention the excessive 'sleep inertia' that results – the grogginess and brain fog that linger long after getting up (see page 27), impacting concentration, mood and even food choices. We don't connect the dots between the grogginess and the lie-in we chose to have – we simply blame our sleep instead.

What if I said it's a trap?

What if I told you that lying in, when it becomes a habit, teaches your brain to stay in limbo? Half-awake, half-asleep, never fully alert. Not because your sleep was bad, but because your system never got the clear signal to switch on.

Now, I promise you: I am not a robot. I have a husband who snores, two businesses to run, a household to run with pets, I lead an NHS sleep service and I'm currently pregnant. I don't have a luxury wellness schedule. What I do have is a morning routine that gives my body the consistency it needs, so I don't spend every weekend recovering or chasing energy.

It doesn't mean I never have bad nights. It means I've taught my body when it's time to be awake. And that consistency? It actually strengthens my sleep from the ground up.

This isn't about being perfect. It's about giving your body one less confusing signal to deal with, so you don't need to lie in, and don't feel like you're constantly recovering from life.

Prescribed 'Sleep-Inducing' Evening Routines Don't Work

Evening relaxation routines alone do not fix sleep problems.

Let's be clear here: I'm not about to say that relaxation and having some 'me time' before bed is bad for you. In fact, research shows that having this 'buffer zone' in your day is valuable. Studies indicate that unwinding before bed can reduce levels of the stress hormone, cortisol, helping the body prepare physiologically for sleep. It gives your mind a chance to slow down and process your day, rather than racing at a million miles an hour right before bed. When anxiety or overthinking take over, they literally shift the chemicals in your brain, with neurotransmitters like dopamine (a stimulating hormone, which isn't what you need right before bed!) disrupting the natural winding-down process your body is designed to go through. Our society is rapidly changing with the acceleration in technology, but we have not rapidly accelerated, meaning we still haven't evolved to deal better with the cognitive overload. When our prehistoric ancestors went to sleep, they didn't even have the same amount of information as a single Netflix episode to process from the day, let alone a whole day of staring at screens and taking in copious amounts of information. So, it makes sense that we do focus on 'winding down' before bed.

The issue is, much like the lie-in paradox, we've been fed another partial truth wrapped up in a comforting package. The commercial sleep industry has popularized the idea that a rigid evening routine is essential, but this just isn't supported by the science. There's a reason we see endless products and apps promoting themselves as 'sleep tools' – they set up our expectations. We think that the more tools, rituals or gadgets we have, the better we'll sleep. But here's the science: these tools don't reset or create the sleep drive your body needs to sleep deeply and consistently. By marketing relaxation and anxiety tools as 'sleep solutions', these products reinforce a belief that isn't entirely true (we will talk about other gadgets in Chapter 7).

It's true that winding down and reducing stress can

help us avoid interrupting the natural sleep process, but relaxation doesn't directly impact the core biological processes that control when and how well you sleep. This is where the real science kicks in. Picture your body clock and sleep drive as two powerful engines driving your sleep needs. No amount of peaceful, quiet time will make these engines work as they should. Relaxation helps prepare you mentally, but it's not turning those engines on; it's merely smoothing the way.

Focusing solely on evening sleep routines as the most important thing will send you spinning in circles. Commercial sleep aids have unintentionally led us to believe that the right bedtime routine is a solution in itself, but what it often does is keep us obsessively trying to control every detail of our night. This turns that lovely 'buffer zone' between wake time and sleep time into more of a 'buffer burden'. Obsessing over 'sleep rituals' often adds more stress, which can then increase cortisol levels and delay sleep further, leaving you in a loop of trying and failing. When you're convinced that your sleep depends on a strict set of rituals, it's easy to feel out of control the moment those rituals aren't met.

Without a well-aligned body clock and a properly built sleep drive over time, even the most serene pre-sleep ritual can only take you so far. It's like sitting in a car with the engine off, adjusting the mirrors and wondering why you're not moving. If you want predictable, restorative sleep, start by prioritizing the body clock and sleep drive, and let relaxation be what it was meant to be – a helpful but secondary part of your day. Besides, it would be nice to still sleep when you don't have time for elaborate relaxation routines, wouldn't it? It's a good thing that's something your body can do, if you know how! Stick to relaxation for the purposes of just that – relaxing. Take away the notion that it will make you sleep and suddenly it becomes a helpful tool again.

Why Your Body Clock and Sleep Drive Rule Everything

Your body clock and sleep drive, which we discussed in Part 1, work together to time and coordinate your sleep needs, but they're obsessed with one thing: consistency. For sleep to work as it's supposed to, it's when you sleep that matters most, over time. It's not just about how many hours you got last night or how relaxed you were; true rest relies on a regular pattern in your behaviour that your body comes to expect.

Changing your sleep timing regularly – whether by trying to get extra hours with an early bedtime or 'catching up' on weekends with a lie-in – doesn't just throw off sleep, it impacts nearly everything the body does within that twenty-four-hour cycle. Appetite, mood, body temperature – all of these rely on that steady rhythm set by your body clock. Imagine that each time you adjust your wake time, it's like shifting gears on a well-oiled machine. One small change throws off the whole system, and your body's left struggling to keep up, unsure if it should be awake, sleepy, hungry or ready to rest.

Picture your internal clock like a meticulous, time-obsessed manager. Every time you shift the routine, the controller scrambles, trying to recalibrate the entire system. Your body expects you to be awake, perhaps already having breakfast or moving around, but, instead, you're lying in bed. So, cortisol, appetite-regulating hormones, energy levels and a bunch of other processes all go haywire, leaving your body confused. Suddenly, by bedtime, you're wondering why sleep seems so far off and why you're wide awake right when you want to wind down.

Meanwhile, the sleep drive – like a battery that gradually charges as the day goes on – gets thrown off balance when you lie in. If you don't let it fully charge, you're left with a half-charged battery that doesn't have enough energy to carry you through the night without disruptions. This isn't about an occasional lie-in or early night. Of course, I occasionally stay up late or enjoy a lazy morning. The difference is that, most of the time, I stick to a routine, so the occasional change doesn't throw me off balance. But if you look at your patterns and see constant shifts or a different weekend routine, that's when sleep quality breaks down. That's when you experience unrefreshing sleep, groggy mornings and rest that feels more like a patchwork than a full recharge.

Your body craves consistency, just like any habit, and when it doesn't get it, sleep quality pays the price. This is why I've seen from experience – and from science – that focusing on *when* we sleep, not just how much or how relaxed we feel, is the key to truly repairing broken sleep.

You don't need to go to bed at the same time every night

You might be thinking or have been advised: I have to go to bed at the same time every night. But haven't you tried that already? Haven't you spent nights lying in bed, 'willing' sleep to come, only to be kept awake by a racing mind? Lying there, thinking about everything from overdue emails to that random song stuck in your head – sound familiar? This is your brain trying to fill the void, left alone in the dark, without the cues it needs for rest. And it makes sense – if you're not the right kind of tired, with the right kind of sleep drive built up, you are not, no matter how much you will it to be, going to fall asleep. You can be a zen-like monk with your relaxation and mindfulness skills, but it is not going to happen. So, if you aren't supposed to have a rigid evening routine, go to bed at the same time or early, or lie in... what on earth are you to do?!

Your Morning Routine Toolkit

Let's course-correct and focus on strategies that actually support your body clock and sleep drive, which, in turn, answers your real question: how do I get to sleep and how do I sleep through the night more consistently?

Have a regular get-up time

I know you don't want me to say it, because of the heavy indoctrination we have into lying in and 'recovering' or 'relaxing', but hear me out. You simply would not feel this way if the majority of your behaviour patterns were set, or 'anchored', by that first one – the get-up time. If there was one thing I could ask everyone on this planet to try – and they couldn't do anything else to manage their sleep – it would be to have a regular get-up time. I often say, if you want to fix your sleep, you have to focus on being awake. This starts in the morning.

Now, I do appreciate that when you have broken sleep already or have had a really bad night, it seems counter-intuitive to start by getting up rather than lying in. But this only seems counter-intuitive because your logic is that a good night's sleep starts in the evening, when you now know that it starts in the morning. And, if you want to change it, you have to start at the right place. If you're reading this thinking, 'But how am I supposed to do that when I feel so groggy in the morning?', remember that most worthwhile things are indeed a bit harder at the beginning. That's why I'm going to give you some additional 'booster'-style strategies to add to your morning to make this whole process easier, quickly. Before we do that though, let's understand why simply focusing on get-up time is the answer.

It all comes down to the power of circadian rhythms. When you get up at the same time each day, you're setting a daily anchor for your body clock, which stabilizes your internal rhythm and allows all other processes to follow a predictable pattern. This stability promotes a smoother sleep–wake cycle, so you're likely to feel alert in the morning and naturally ready for bed in the evening, regardless of slight shifts or disruptions that might impact your bedtime. That's right – in order to feel more sleepy at the right times, to get you through the night, you need to focus on being awake, which starts in the morning.

Unlike bedtime, which can fluctuate depending on life's events or emotional and physical factors, your wake-up time provides a consistent signal that your body can reliably organize around. But let's be clear: I'm not just talking about *waking* up when your alarm goes off. I'm talking about *getting* up – getting out of bed, exposing yourself to light and moving. Just lying in bed with your eyes open doesn't count. Your body clock needs clear signals, and those only come when you get out of bed and start the day. It's the difference between tapping snooze and confusing your system, or getting up and telling your brain: 'It's morning – let's go.'

This is why I start sleep treatment for my clients with this strategy (just like Suli), rather than focusing on anything else that might 'aid' sleep. Without starting with a regular get-up time, varying sleep times can lead to feeling jet-lagged, where the body clock is constantly recalibrating, resulting in grogginess, lowered energy and unstable sleep – and by unstable, I mean constantly struggling to actually sleep, whether that be at the beginning of the night or in the middle/towards the end. Bedtime will become more predictable, and it's likely you will start to feel like you can go to sleep at around the same time (the idea that you can take yourself to bed at the same time every day if you aren't looking after your morning routine is utterly pointless). Also, you're very likely to kill that 'tired but wired' feeling that you might get at bedtime, which you might be desperately trying to resolve. It could be that your sleep drive is not strong or predictable enough.

Trust me, once you have nailed your morning routine, you will be surprised at all the positive effects – even before we have resolved their entire sleep issue, my clients feel better for it, rather than worse. But I know that means having to get into the rhythm of things, and to start with it's always a touch harder. Back to those helpful 'boosts' that are going to help you regain the art of a good morning routine:

Get more light

Expose yourself to light as soon as you can at get-up time – even after a bad night of sleep, light can improve how alert you feel and lift your mood. It's like a superpower – imagine all the positive effects of coffee times ten with none of the negatives! Light is so powerful we can even use it in a timed fashion as treatment in certain sleep disorders where the sleep timing is off.

The reason light is so influential on our circadian rhythm is simple: our bodies evolved to respond to the Earth's natural light and dark cycles. For billions of years, life on this planet has been shaped by the twenty-four-hour rotation of the Earth, giving us predictable cycles of day and night. And over millions of years, humans adapted to these cycles too. We aren't completely aligned though (and it's helpful to have a bit of adaptability, such as for when we change time zones), so light helps us stay on track.

Our bodies have a 'master clock' located in the brain's hypothalamus called the suprachiasmatic nucleus (or SCN, for short), which keeps time for all sorts of processes in the body. This master clock relies heavily on cues from light. Specifically, when morning light hits your eyes, it signals the SCN to wake things up – just like an alarm clock. Cortisol, our natural 'get-up-and-go' hormone (it's not just a stress hormone – I prefer to refer to it as a wake hormone), starts flowing, and melatonin (the hormone that makes us sleepy) gets switched off. It's like a daily reset, aligning our body clock with the twenty-four-hour day so we're in sync with our environment. It also means that light is incredibly useful when suffering from jet lag – the sooner you get light when the locals in your new time zone do, rather than avoiding the day because you're exhausted, the sooner you'll transition.

How to get more light for better sleep

- Get outside as soon as you can after waking.
- Aim for ten to thirty minutes of light exposure (even on cloudy days).
- Use a 10,000 lux light box or a wake-up light if needed, or even just bright artificial light if that's all you can do (if you don't have access to natural light).

Remember: morning light = better sleep at night.

This isn't just about feeling awake – it's about staying on track. Light anchors your body clock. Daylight helps us feel alert and energetic, while darkness prepares us for rest. The problem? Modern life has thrown this natural rhythm off balance. With artificial light everywhere, our poor SCN is confused. Evening exposure to things like phones, TV screens and overhead bright lights, tricks it into thinking it's still daytime, which can mess with our sleep and delay the natural release of melatonin.

If you've ever wondered why morning light feels like a boost while screens at night leave you wired, this is why. We evolved to depend on light as a natural cue to stay aligned with the Earth's rhythms. That's why light is such a powerful influence on our internal clock and why it plays a huge role in regulating our sleep, mood and energy. You may have even noticed that, after some particularly rainy days, a bit of sunshine can 'lift' you. It also means that after a few days of getting used to it, sleeping in nature, away from technology, can really improve your sleep quality and how you feel during the day.

Natural light is like the gold standard for resetting your body clock. It's brighter and richer in the blue light wavelengths that are particularly effective at waking us up, signalling to our brains that it's time to be alert and active. Plus, it changes gradually throughout the day, reinforcing cues for energy in the morning and slowing us down as evening sets in. So, get outside whenever you can. Even if it's just for ten minutes in the morning or on a coffee break, getting natural light exposure – even on cloudy days – can help. Aim for early-morning light, if possible, as this is most effective for setting your circadian rhythm.

Let's face it, though, many of us spend our days indoors, surrounded by artificial light that just doesn't cut it. Office lights, phone screens and even LED bulbs simply aren't bright enough to send that strong 'daytime' signal.

And if you live somewhere with long winters or cloudy skies, you're definitely not getting enough natural light to keep your body clock on track. To be honest, I would say, whatever your level of light is, you likely need a bit more in your mornings especially.

So, what can you do? Here are a few next best things to natural light:

- Light therapy lamps. These lamps mimic natural sunlight and are especially useful in the darker months or if you have a schedule that keeps you inside. Place one on your desk or use it in the morning for about twenty to thirty minutes. Look for lamps with at least 10,000 lux (that's the level needed to simulate sunlight).
- Wake-up light alarms. These alarms gradually brighten your room, simulating a sunrise that gently cues your body to wake up. It's a much kinder way to start the day than a blaring alarm and helps you wake up in a lighter stage of sleep.
- Blue-enriched light bulbs. For those really struggling with dark mornings or office lighting, there are specially designed light bulbs that emit more blue-spectrum light. Use them during the day to help signal 'daytime' to your body clock.

A couple of hours before bed, try to reduce the lighting and brightness of devices too. This not only dials down that wavelength of blue light which seems to be so effective, but I also don't want to encourage the use of tech before bed, because usually it's a source of information, and the evening is not the time to be introducing yet more information for our brains to process when really we want to wind down. Limiting use of or dimming overhead lights and screens one to two hours before bed is a step in the right direction.

Light is powerful. It is not the same as any other 'supplements' or tech you hear of that has been sold to you as a sleep aid. This is real and, besides, most of the time, it's free!

Don't just lie there... move!

Here's the lowdown on why getting up and moving first thing, instead of just lying in bed, is a game-changer for your energy levels, mood and sleep–wake cycle: when you get up and get moving in the morning, you're sending your body strong signals that 'It's time to wake up.'

Movement works in tandem with light exposure to reinforce your body's natural rhythm. Here's how it all works:

- Boosting cortisol (in a good way). Morning movement helps release cortisol, which we now understand to be your body's natural 'wake-up' hormone. This is cortisol doing what it's supposed to do, giving you energy and alertness to start the day. Lying in bed, on the other hand, doesn't give the body this same 'wake-up' signal, so you're more likely to feel sluggish and unmotivated.

- Improving mood. Movement releases endorphins, those feel-good hormones that naturally boost your mood. Even gentle movement, like stretching or a short walk, can lower stress levels and make you feel more positive. So, instead of lying there thinking about how tired you are, you're physically priming yourself to feel good and ready for the day.
- Syncing the body clock. Getting up and moving also helps set your internal clock, or circadian rhythm, in sync with the day. Morning movement combined with light exposure tells your body that the day has started, helping you stay more alert in the morning and naturally wind down at night. This rhythm leads to better energy during the day and more restorative sleep at night.
- Building energy (instead of draining it). It sounds counter-intuitive, but movement actually builds energy and reduces fatigue. When you move, your circulation improves and more oxygen reaches your cells, making you feel

more alert. Lying in bed has the opposite effect – your body stays in that low-energy 'sleep mode' which often makes you feel even more tired and groggy.

In short, getting up and moving first thing is like giving your body the green light to switch into 'awake mode', setting you up for better energy, mood and sleep quality. You don't have to fit in your entire exercise regime for the day. Even twenty minutes of stretching, walking the dog or doing a free online exercise routine would help you. So, next time you wake up, don't just lie there – get up, get moving and let your body do what it's designed to do.

Keep to consistent mealtimes (even if you're not a breakfast person)

This might seem like an odd addition, but it's a good one. Without diving into the diet wars, because we all know people have strong feelings about their meal choices, whether it's keto, intermittent fasting or skipping breakfast entirely – we're not here to argue the merits of what you eat. But we are here to talk about when you eat and why keeping to consistent mealtimes can actually help support your energy, mood and sleep.

So, here's the deal: have some regularity around your eating times. Here's why it helps:

- 🕐 Body clock consistency. Just like light and movement, eating sends strong signals to your internal clock – it is a 'time keeper'. Our bodies have these mini clocks, especially in the digestive system, that rely on regular mealtimes to stay in sync with our rhythm.
- 🕐 Consistent energy and alertness levels. Eating at regular times helps keep your energy steady throughout the day. When you eat whenever (or skip meals), you're more likely to go through 'highs' and 'lows', where you feel full of energy one minute and sluggish the next. But a regular eating pattern gives you a steady supply of fuel, so you're less likely to feel those midday slumps or late-afternoon dips. It's about keeping things balanced, not obsessing over every snack.
- 🕐 Better sleep–wake signals. Here's the kicker – your body clock actually notices when you eat, and it uses that information to help time your sleep–wake cycle. If you're all over the place with mealtimes, it can throw off the body's sense of 'day' versus 'night'. But if you keep things regular, you're giving your body another solid anchor for knowing when it's time to be awake and when it's time to rest.
- 🕐 Mood stability. Consistent eating times also stabilize your mood. Without the hangry dips, you're less likely to snap at everyone in your way

or feel that irritable low-energy slump. It's like giving your mood a smooth runway to stay level.

Having some sort of breakfast helps you start this cycle off after your overnight fast, and I have two things to say about this. Firstly, I understand that not everyone is into breakfast, so, like I say, having some consistency in the mealtimes *you choose to have* will be better than no consistency – it's just the more your behaviours are in line with when your body naturally wants to be awake (i.e. the morning), the more predictable things like your sleep, mood and energy become. Secondly, be sure that you haven't just trained yourself not to feel hungry for breakfast. Your brain is smart and it will take hunger cues away if it knows, quite predictably, that there is a different time of day when it will first be fed (hunger can be predictive, not just reactive!). We always feel we are responding to our bodily processes, but your brain is often one step ahead, adapting your bodily processes to your behaviours.

So, whether you're a breakfast fanatic or someone who can't even look at food till noon, try to keep your meal schedule regular. A bit of consistency works wonders on your body clock, giving you better energy, focus and even sleep in the long run.

Choose an alarm that works for you, not against you

It's true that being jolted awake by a loud alarm, especially when you're deep in sleep, can feel unpleasant. Research suggests that sudden auditory alarms can activate the sympathetic nervous system (the fight-or-flight response), leading to increased heart rate, blood pressure and a temporary stress response. This might be particularly problematic if you're already vulnerable to cardiovascular conditions or experiencing chronic sleep deprivation.

But here's the nuance that often gets missed: most of these studies don't differentiate between people with regular sleep habits and a strong sleep baseline, and those who are sleep-deprived or have unpredictable sleep patterns – using alarms when needed for work and then not at all any other time. In other words, we don't really know how harmful alarms are in the context of already consistent, healthy sleep. And this is key, because context always matters.

So, yes, snoozing for thirty minutes with constant micro-awakenings might confuse your brain and body, giving mixed signals to your circadian system. But using an alarm to anchor your get-up time while you're rebuilding that baseline? That's not harmful – it's essential. It gives your brain a stable cue, which helps regulate the sleep–wake cycle over time.

Ideally, once your sleep drive and body clock are

better aligned, you'll wake naturally before your alarm goes off sometimes. But while you're getting there, don't be afraid to use one – just be strategic. Light, movement and consistent mealtimes will start helping your body become more predictable – and that means in the future feeling ready to get up before you do these things! But, in the short term, to get you through the tough bit while your old patterns and groggy feelings in the morning are still in your system, try these tricks:

- Keep your alarm out of arm's reach. This is the classic, and for good reason. If your alarm's right next to your bed, half-asleep-you will just slap that snooze button without a second thought. So, put it across the room. Now, to turn it off, you actually have to get out of bed. And once you're up, you're far less likely to crawl back in.
- Try the 'double alarm' trick. Set one alarm across the room to get you up, then another one in the bathroom or kitchen. Now you're basically forcing yourself into a little morning scavenger hunt. By the time you find the second alarm and turn it off, you're already halfway to starting your day and it stops you lying in bed for too long once you're awake. Eventually, your body will sync with these cues and you will notice you naturally feel like getting up anyway!

❹ Invest in a light alarm. This is my personal favourite – I have one and I will never go back. They don't wake you abruptly like noise alarms do. Instead, light alarms mimic a natural sunrise and ease you out of sleep more gently, reducing that cortisol spike and grogginess. (You can set a noise if you really want to, for the end, just to be sure – but maybe make it a more pleasant one!)

Your New Sleep Strategy

Picture this: you get up early every weekday but indulge in lie-ins on weekends. This pattern throws off your body's rhythm, so, by Sunday night, you're wide awake and dreading Monday morning. They call them the 'Sunday night blues'... But your new routine will likely resolve all this!

Your new alternatives to obsessive night-time rituals, going to bed when you're not tired and lying in, can now start when sleep processes truly start: with your morning routine, by getting up, getting light, moving your body and having consistent mealtimes that work for you. Eventually, you will notice a more consistent bedtime as you start to feel sleepier more predictably, and you can also limit the amount of light and information you consume in those hours before bed to help facilitate the process, without overly obsessing about it. Because the window of your sleep becomes more consistent, and your body reliably knows when you are going to hit the hay and get up, you will also notice the quality of sleep and any gaps in your sleep improving (though, when things have become very broken, such as when we get sleep disorders, further treatment is required, and we will discuss this in the appendix – page 273).

Your morning routine reset!

If you're going to change one thing, let it be your morning. Here's a recap of your simple, powerful routine to reset your sleep – starting from the moment you wake up:

- Get up at the same time every day, even on weekends. This anchors your body clock and builds a predictable sleep window. You want to actually *get up* within ten minutes or less!

- Get light ASAP. Natural daylight is ideal (within thirty to sixty minutes of waking), even on cloudy days. A lightbox can help in winter.

- Move your body. Even gentle movement like stretching, walking the dog or a light workout helps wake you up and boosts mood and energy.

- Stick to regular mealtimes. Try to eat at around the same times each day, even if breakfast is not your thing. Your body clock uses food timing to stay in sync.

- Dial down the pressure on bedtime. Let sleep come to you. Go to bed when you're tired and not before – this will happen more predictably when you have nailed your morning routine. Skip the rigid wind-down rituals and focus on winding your day down, not forcing sleep to arrive.

This is your foundation. Nail this first. If you're doing even just some of this, more often than not, you're building a stronger sleep baseline – and that will always serve you more than any supplement, gadget or miracle routine.

At first, Suli was sceptical about the idea that her mornings mattered more than her evenings. Her nightly routine was a carefully curated ritual of herbal teas, relaxation apps, warm baths and rigid bedtimes. But, despite her best efforts, sleep wasn't cooperating. When I introduced her to the concept of focusing on morning habits instead, she was willing to give it a try.

The first step was committing to a consistent get-up time – even on weekends. This was tough at first, especially after a restless night, but we paired it with light exposure and gentle movement to jump-start her mornings. Suli started taking her dogs for a quick morning walk as soon as she got up, even when it was overcast or a bit darker (she made sure the lights were bright at home). To her surprise, she found the fresh air and light lifted her grogginess far better than lying in.

We also worked on reducing her reliance on evening rituals. Instead of obsessing over her nightly 'wind-down' routine, Suli shifted her focus to the simplicity of her mornings. Within just a few weeks, her sleep patterns began to stabilize. She reported feeling naturally sleepy at night without forcing it – even her constant overthinking and rise in anxiety was dulled by the sleepiness without having to directly target it – and waking up feeling more refreshed. While this is not all we can do to resolve a chronic sleep problem, for Suli, it was indeed all she needed.

Suli is doing very well still. She told me: 'Over a couple of months, I went from getting one hour's sleep a night to five or six. Now, six months later, I get around six or seven. I genuinely don't perceive myself to be a poor sleeper anymore – it's life after insomnia for me. The difference is now I don't worry about a few nights of poor sleep (because it always turns back around) and I know how to take care of my sleep in general, which makes me feel more in control. I can't believe all the things I would add in to my day in the hope it would make me sleep – it seems so simple now. And I have more energy! I've joined loads more social activities. I can see more of my friends. In short: I have a life again.' (Coming from Suli, who was already very busy, this is quite the win!)

Suli's story shows just how powerful these foundations can be – and how even after years of broken sleep, things can turn around.

Consistency Is the Formula for Good Sleep

I'm not saying you have to be an angel and stick perfectly to your new routine every single day (though, if you did, even just for a few weeks as an experiment, you'd notice how much better you feel). I get that being 100 per cent consistent isn't always realistic. But let's take out some of those old excuses – like regularly trying to 'catch up' on sleep, dragging out the morning because you don't feel like getting up or having wildly different get-up times. Those habits just leave your body clock completely confused.

If you could just improve your consistency with a regular get-up more often than you don't, rather than trying to be perfect, you will likely notice a difference. According to research, people with consistent wake times across the week tend to report higher sleep quality and are significantly less likely to experience symptoms of insomnia, even if their total sleep time isn't longer. That's how powerful a more regular get-up routine can be.

I've said it before and I'll say it again: what I'm teaching you in this book is not the same as all the other advice, gadgets, drugs and supplements, and any other magical solutions you can think of out there for your sleep. These are the fundamentals, meaning they are the most influential – and if you do happen to find a supplement or hack which has some sliver of evidence to actually improve your sleep (something we will explore in Chapter 7), they won't even touch the sides if these fundamentals aren't in place first. Use your time, energy, attention and money wisely.

Sometimes sleep just won't go your way

Sure, there are going to be times when you wake up earlier than planned, or your sleep's more broken, or you just lie there with your mind racing (despite your now much better efforts!). We talked about this back in Chapter 1 – life throws in sleep disruptors like stress, illness, hormonal changes, chronic conditions, pregnancy and, yes, just getting older. But these aren't the norm, and if we were taught from a young age to support our body clocks, they'd have less impact anyway. Let's focus on what we can control, because we can't do much about the rest.

This is especially key for anyone dealing with big life variations like chronic health issues, which can affect everything from sleep and mood to appetite and body temperature (all controlled by your trusty body clock). So, let's give ourselves a head start: a solid baseline makes it easier to handle these curveballs when they come (and we will talk about learning the joy of imperfect sleep and managing our expectations in Part 3).

In this chapter, we've cleared up some common misconceptions and replaced them with practical, science-backed strategies that can reshape how you approach sleep. To help you along the way, keep these key points in mind:

- When you sleep can be more influential than obsessing over how much you sleep. Focusing on timing, not duration, gives you more control over quality rest.
- Stick to the core principles of sleep, not myths, trends or 'logical' fixes. Sleep science debunks many popular ideas. Building habits around what actually works will help far more than trying the latest sleep fad.
- Think long term. Consistency is the secret. What you do over weeks, not just what happened last night, will make sleep serve you predictably and effectively.
- You don't have to be perfect. Healthy habits work best when they're part of a flexible routine, not rigid rules. Even doing them more often than not will make a difference. The goal isn't perfection but rather developing reliable routines that put sleep back on your side.

Even when you're doing everything right, things can still go off course sometimes and you end up lying in bed wide awake. And it's not always sleep itself that's the problem. It's the thoughts – the mental to-do list; the random memories; the rising panic that you're awake when you 'should' be asleep. This is where so many people get stuck – not just because sleep is fragile, but because their thoughts have started running the show.

In the next chapter, we're going to talk about what happens when your brain won't shut up at the worst possible time – and how to stop those thoughts from hijacking your nights.

CHAPTER 5

Tired But Wired: Meet the Sleep Anxiety Gremlins

The problem: Sleep anxiety – the fear of not sleeping – can spiral into a vicious cycle that disrupts sleep further.

The fix: Build a strong sleep baseline, learn how to respond to anxious thoughts in the moment and reframe your mindset so sleep no longer feels like something to control.

You've been here before, haven't you? The lights are off, the room is quiet, but your brain... your brain is anything but. You're thinking, 'What if I don't sleep at all tonight?' Then, 'If I don't fall asleep soon, tomorrow will be ruined.' And the *pièce de résistance*: 'What if I never sleep properly again?' These thoughts aren't new. They're as familiar as the pattern on your duvet, and they never lead anywhere good. Some of these thoughts are regular visitors, while others creep in after days or weeks of disrupted sleep. Sometimes, it's not even sleep itself you're anxious about – it's overthinking, work or life.

The Gremlins in the Dark

It's worth knowing that your brain isn't wired to be rational in the middle of the night. In fact, we're neurologically more prone to threat-based thinking during the night, especially when half-awake. Your brain is in 'threat detection mode' – a leftover from when being alert at night was essential for survival. That's why, in the early hours, everything feels bigger, scarier and more dramatic. Have you ever reflected on your night-time thoughts in the morning? You will be surprised at some of the things that no longer feel rational! We are not supposed to be using our brains the way we do during the day, at night-time. We are just not good at it.

You might not even be thinking about sleep at all to begin with – just worrying about your job, your family or something you said three weeks ago; you even might be buzzing from a good day! It's only once your mind has gone down that rabbit hole for a while that you then start panicking about the fact you're awake, or at least very frustrated because you came to bed to sleep. It's important to acknowledge this: not all night-time anxiety starts with sleep.

However, once the general night-time worry or overthinking kicks off, it often *does* turn its attention to sleep. After all, you're lying in bed, you're aware that time is passing and you've been taught that sleep is both essential and fragile. So, your brain, in its overprotective late-night state, latches on to the next 'logical' fear: *What if I don't sleep?* That's when the real sleep anxiety gremlins show up, and they're clever little devils. They wait until everything else is calm, then creep in and take over your head. But don't be fooled – these thoughts aren't harmless musings. They change your brain chemistry. They turn on your cortisol, flooding your body with a hormone that's meant to wake you up and get you moving in the morning, not lull you to sleep. Worse, they suppress melatonin, your natural sleep hormone, as if pulling the rug out from under you just as you're trying to relax. You essentially flick a switch and voila – you have pushed sleep away.

And what happens next? You panic. You try everything: counting sheep, switching pillows, changing rooms and scrolling through every sleep hack Google has to offer. Maybe you turn to sleeping pills or wine, desperately trying to force sleep to come. But these behaviours don't work in the way you think they will. Instead of helping, they send one loud, clear message to your brain: *I can't sleep on my own.* And the gremlins? They love this. This call to action fuels them harder, rather than quietening them down.

Sleep anxiety gremlins have two weapons

1. They can change your brain chemistry – so it's not just unhelpful thinking... very quickly, they can literally push sleep away.

2. They convince you to change your behaviour to bring sleep back – you need instant results *now* and so you become their puppet, not necessarily choosing the healthiest behaviours, and therefore making sleep worse.

The self-fulfilling cycle of sleep anxiety

Here's the thing: the fear of not sleeping can be worse than not sleeping itself. I see this all the time in clinic, and the research backs it up. Studies have shown that people who believe they are insomniacs often experience worse daytime fatigue, mood and health outcomes than those who objectively sleep poorly but don't label themselves that way. Psychologist Kenneth Lichstein and others have described this as a kind of *insomnia identity*, where the worry about poor sleep can often do more damage than the sleep loss itself. Read that again. The belief that you're broken can be more damaging than the sleep loss.

It's not just perception – it's biology. When you stress about sleep or anything else, especially at night, your body produces more cortisol and adrenaline. This

Worry about poor sleep can often do more damage than the sleep loss itself.

Harm caused

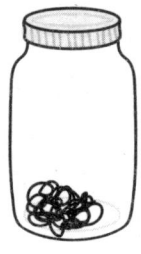
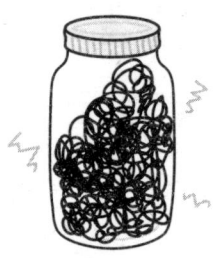

Experiencing poor sleep   Worrying about poor sleep

'fight-or-flight' response evolved to keep you alive in moments of danger, like escaping a predator. But in bed, there are no predators – just your thoughts, convincing your body it's in crisis. Elevated cortisol levels can affect everything from your heart rate to your digestive system. It's why you feel tense, jittery and alert when all you want is to rest. Your body can't tell the difference between a tiger and a ticking clock.

    And how we think about sleep matters just as much as the sleep itself. Let's take two hypothetical people. One sleeps poorly and feels perfectly fine the next day. They might say, 'Ah well, bad sleep happens!' and go about their life. The other sleeps just as poorly but spirals into worry: 'What's wrong with me? Why can't I sleep? How will I get through tomorrow?' The fascinating thing? Despite both having the same poor sleep, their outcomes couldn't be more different.

Research published in the *Journal of Psychosomatic Research* found that individuals who experienced objectively poor sleep but didn't perceive it as a problem were less likely to experience the negative health outcomes often associated with insomnia. These 'non-anxious poor sleepers' had lower levels of daytime fatigue, better mood regulation and fewer symptoms of depression compared to those who worried about their sleep.

Why does this happen? Anxiety amplifies the effects of poor sleep. When you're anxious about not sleeping, you create a cascade of physiological and psychological responses: elevated cortisol, increased heart rate and, of course, more worrying thoughts. All of these feed into the sleep–worry–sleep cycle, making it harder for your body to recover.

So, what makes the difference? It's perception. When you believe your sleep is 'broken' or feel that it's something you must fix immediately, you add layers of stress that wouldn't otherwise exist. Think of it this way: sleep anxiety isn't just an extra layer on top of poor sleep – it's an amplifier. It's the volume knob that cranks up the negative effects of a bad night.

The night before a big event

I once got a message on social media from a man who explained a common theme:

> *I'm a cognitive behavioural professor, and I sleep well now, most of the time. But the night before I have to present in front of a big audience, I just don't sleep well. And I don't know how to handle it.*

You've got a big day tomorrow – a presentation, an interview, a trip, a family event – so you think: 'Right, I need a good night's sleep tonight.' That pressure builds throughout the day. Maybe you even go to bed early, hoping to squeeze in extra rest. But, instead, you lie there – buzzing, alert, irritated. The more you try to sleep, the more it slips away. This is such a common pattern – even I don't sleep the same as usual before big events.

Let's break down why this happens and what actually helps:

- Big day = big pressure. When something important is coming up, your nervous system is already activated – whether it's excitement, anticipation or anxiety – and your physiology shifts: cortisol rises and adrenaline might spike. This isn't 'bad' – it's just your body preparing you for action. But it also means sleep may not come easily.

- Going to bed early often backfires. If you're not truly tired, heading to bed early just stretches the sleep window. You lie in bed longer, thinking more, becoming more frustrated – and creating the perfect storm for fragmented or delayed sleep.

What helps instead? This is exactly what I do:

- Go to bed later, not earlier. If you're wired, it's better to give yourself time to wind down than try to force sleep (but do wind down – don't spend time on your presentation, going over your packing list or anything to do with tomorrow!). You'll likely sleep deeper once you do drift off, even if you sleep a little less.

- Change your expectations. Of course, sleep might look different before a big day – that's normal. It doesn't mean you've regressed. Don't overcorrect. Avoid piling on rituals or routines in a desperate attempt to 'guarantee' sleep. Stick to your baseline habits.

- Reframe the impact. A slightly poorer night of sleep before a big event isn't always harmful. In fact, there's some research suggesting that short-term sleep deprivation can reduce overthinking and inhibition, helping you to focus more clearly and care a little less about what others think – which, for things like public speaking, can actually work in your favour. I often think, 'At least I won't care as much if I'm a bit tired!'

Remember, the goal isn't perfect sleep before every big day. It's resilience. You already know how to sleep. So, even if one night isn't ideal, you've built the foundation to carry you through.

The myth that keeps us awake

Here's where the sleep anxiety gremlins can get even sneakier: they feed off the deeply ingrained myth *I need to control my sleep.* Think about it. What's the first thing you do when you can't sleep? You try to 'fix' it. Maybe you start a new evening routine, adjust your bedtime or obsessively track your sleep with an app. But, as we know now, sleep doesn't work that way. Sleep is not something you can force. It's a natural, self-regulating process controlled by your circadian rhythm and sleep drive. The more you try to control it, the more you disrupt these systems.

Imagine trying to fall asleep while a voice in your head constantly says, 'Sleep! Sleep now! If you don't, tomorrow's ruined!' Would you be able to relax? Of course not. That's what happens when you let the gremlins run the show.

And to add to it all, worrying about sleep doesn't just make you feel more unwell, it can bring on a sleep disorder. Let's return to the science. In another fascinating study from the *Journal of Clinical Sleep Medicine*, researchers found that people with high levels of 'sleep reactivity' (a term for how much stress about sleep impacts their lives) were more likely to develop chronic insomnia. Not because they were sleeping poorly, but because they worried about sleeping poorly.

Worry turns a few bad nights into a self-perpetuating cycle. The gremlins take one bad night and whisper, 'This is just the beginning. It's all downhill from here.' And then you start adjusting everything – your bedtime, your lifestyle (cancelling activities like the gym and

A bad night's sleep

Feels like a disaster in the moment

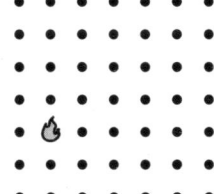

But it's just <u>one</u> dot on a bigger timeline

social engagements), your mindset – trying to regain control. Ironically, all this overcorrecting reinforces the belief that sleep is fragile and out of your control, which only feeds the gremlins more. All of these changes also move you further away from your normal sleep–wake cycle, rather than pushing you towards it.

The Reality Check: What Actually Happens After a 'Bad' Night

Here's something the sleep anxiety gremlins don't want you to know: your body is resilient. After a poor night, your sleep drive increases, making it nearly impossible to stay awake indefinitely. If you've ever pulled an all-nighter, you've felt this – by the next evening, your body practically drags you to bed.

'That doesn't happen to me,' you might say, 'it just gets worse.' There are reasons you feel this way – your sleep baseline is weak, meaning your sleep drive and circadian regulation is so misaligned that this mechanism can't work the way it wants to. If your sleep muscle – the strength and stability of your natural sleep–wake systems – is weak, then building that baseline through regular morning routines, movement, light and consistent patterns (as we saw in the last chapter) can genuinely make a huge difference. For many people, even just starting to work on this can calm the gremlins or even just an active mind at night, because you're giving your body more of the pressure and signals it needs to sleep naturally. You're also proving to yourself that change is possible, and that alone takes the edge off the anxiety.

But I also know this: if your gremlins have grown loud and strong, if sleep anxiety has been around for a while or your anxiety levels are high in general, then even beginning that process can feel impossible. It's like knowing you need to move but feeling too paralysed to take the first step. In those cases, a little extra support is not a failure, it's a smart move. That might mean looking at the sleep disorder section on page 273 to figure out what kind of help is right for you. Whatever your starting point, the work you're doing here lays the foundation – and that foundation is where things start to shift.

And, remember, your brain is also very smart – even when we just can't get out of that anxiety loop, it's still helping you. It adapts by prioritizing the sleep stages it needs most. Missed out on deep sleep? Your body will catch up by increasing slow-wave sleep the next night. Skimped on REM? Expect more vivid dreams as your brain makes up for it. This is the selective rebound we touched on in Chapter 1, and it's your body's way of ensuring you get what you need, even after disruptions.

So, the next time the sleep anxiety gremlins start whispering, 'You're ruining everything by not sleeping,' remind yourself: your body has this under control.

Clock-Watching

There is one thing that deserves an entire section when it comes to those creepy sleep anxiety gremlins. Imagine if, for a third of your day, time simply didn't exist: no ticking hands, no glowing numbers, no reminders of how long you've been awake or how much time is left to sleep. What would that feel like? Liberating? Peaceful? I can tell you it absolutely is! For most of us, checking the clock when we can't sleep feels very automatic. We glance at our phones, our bedside alarms or even the stove clock in a midnight wander. But why? What does it lead to? Does it help you sleep? Does it make you feel better about lying awake? Or does it feed your sleep anxiety gremlins, fuelling thoughts like:

- 🕘 'I've only had four hours of sleep.'
- 🕘 'If I don't fall asleep in the next hour, tomorrow will be a disaster.'
- 🕘 'I'll never catch up on this lost time.'

Clock-watching transforms what could be a restful period of wakefulness into pure stress when we don't even need to know the time! The only time that matters is when your alarm goes off. Everything else is absolutely useless. Clocks, and the way we perceive time, are a human construct, a way of organizing our lives, not a reflection of our biological needs – we have our own clock which doesn't deal in 'perception'. As we learned in Chapter 1, long before clocks existed, people relied on natural cues like light and dark to guide their rhythms. And it worked.

By obsessing over time at night, we impose artificial constraints on our natural sleep process. Sleep doesn't work on a precise schedule; it ebbs and flows according to your circadian rhythms and sleep drive. When we strip away the clock, we free ourselves to trust these innate processes instead of battling them. Remember this next time you're fretting over hours of sleep: your body can do amazing things with twenty minutes of sleep, and you can also toss and turn and have the worst eight hours' sleep of your life! The way we perceive time and what it means is wrong.

When I was assisting in forced desynchrony studies for Harvard Medical School, I had to learn to avoid using any time cues with the subjects. A forced desynchrony protocol was a way of separating the internal sleep mechanisms (our 'master clock') with the external time cues we have around us, like when we eat/move/work/get light and even talk about time (among *many* others). And let me tell you, it was hard. I couldn't say good morning, I couldn't mention what time it was, I couldn't allude to anything that might give the subject a clue of whether it was day or night, Saturday or Thursday or what I ate for my last meal. Try it yourself – have a conversation without alluding to anything which might give away the time to the other person. Ask them to stop you every time they could infer some sort of timing, from the time of day or night, the day of the week or which season we might be in.

It was an important lesson for me. I learned how much my life was governed by time! It also made me want to start liberating myself from it when it wasn't needed, like at night. During the day, time keeps us moving forward and getting things done. At night, it seems to freeze us and nothing gets done. Least of all sleep. As long as I had my alarm set to the same time, my night could play out in whatever way and it wouldn't matter what time I happened to wake or not be able to sleep. I now live in the comfort that it's still some sort of night-time and that, even if all I got was another five minutes of sleep or, indeed, I just rested, I was in a place where time meant nothing at all; I didn't have to think about it until my day started. It really is a comforting, freeing feeling. Try it. The sleep anxiety gremlins especially hate this trick because it disarms their weapons. You may not have won the battles previously, but you are now winning the war.

Tools to Silence the Sleep Anxiety Gremlins

Now that we've exposed their tricks, let's talk about how to fight back! But, first, I need to be really honest about something: there's no single magic cure for sleep anxiety. I wish I could give everyone a one-size-fits-all solution, but, the truth is, managing sleep anxiety is a process – and that process will look slightly different for everyone. For some people, it starts with education – learning how sleep really works and unpicking the myths they've been taught. Then it's about providing themselves with proof that alternative sleep behaviours (keeping your sleep muscle strong by improving your sleep baseline) can impact their sleep positively, which often reduces anxiety all by itself. For others, it's about calming the body in the moment or shifting unhelpful behaviours/thoughts. And, sometimes, it's about distraction – giving the mind something else to hold on to while the body finds its way back to rest, or actively challenging those thoughts. Mostly, it's a combination, and finally getting to that point of realization – sleep will be there regardless of how you treat it, what it looks like or where you are in life. We don't have the ability to just lose it, even though that is often the biggest fear of all.

You don't need to figure it all out at once. The goal is to build your own toolkit and find what combination works best for you. But all of it begins with one mindset shift: stop chasing sleep, and start supporting it. That's where the change happens.

Note: sometimes, anxiety can be so strong that, even though you *know* it's caused by broken sleep, for example, resolving the sleep issues in the way you need to – even with evidence-based insomnia treatment as we describe in the appendix – may not be enough. It may be that you do need some general support with anxiety, such as therapy or medication, at least in the short term. I'm not trying to fob you off here, it's just sometimes you need a few tools to calm it right down before you can even begin to break down the sleep part of the problem and get it resolved for good.

Gremlin triage: your middle-of-the-night survival kit

Let's be clear: these aren't tricks to 'make' you fall asleep. They're tools to calm down the brain, interrupt the anxiety spiral and help your body feel safe enough to do what it naturally knows how to do. Think of them as middle-of-the-night triage – a gentle way to take the pressure off, shift your attention and give your system a chance to reset.

- Reframe wakefulness as rest. Lying awake isn't failure. It's still a form of rest – and your body can benefit from this downtime even if sleep isn't happening. Try saying to yourself: 'I'm resting, and that's enough for now.'
- Plan for wakefulness. If you're not asleep after a while, at the beginning of the night, in the middle or even just an hour before your usual get-up time, don't stay in bed getting more worked up. Gently leave the bed (or just sit somewhere different in the room) and do something low-stimulus but absorbing that is more in line with your evening routine – like reading, journaling or listening to music or a podcast. You might even consider setting aside a few things in advance – a book you enjoy, a calming playlist, a notebook – so you don't have to make decisions in the middle of the night, which can be stressful. I call this creating your 'bonus time' kit. The idea is not to entertain yourself too much, but to lower the mental effort and take the pressure off. Try not to just 'get up earlier' to start your day either if it's not just a one off – you will train your brain into getting up earlier!

- Challenge the gremlins. When those spiralling thoughts kick in – 'I'll never cope tomorrow' – talk back. Remind yourself of the evidence: 'I've had bad nights before, and I managed just fine.' And be honest: how often have you predicted your day would be awful... and it wasn't? How often were you fired/made massive errors? I bet way less than you have feared it – if at all!
- Zoom out. One night is just one dot on a much bigger timeline. You're not aiming for perfect sleep every night – you're building patterns over weeks. Remind yourself: 'This one night doesn't define anything.'

'In-the-moment' techniques to reduce anxiety

There are many tools you can use in the moment to calm down racing thoughts and anxiety – from breathwork to body scan techniques, distraction and imagery techniques. You likely will need to find something which truly resonates with you that you can practise at any time of the day to become confident and positive that it makes you feel better. I always find a good place to get inspiration is free YouTube videos – save them once you have found ones that might work for you. When you stop trying to force sleep and focus instead on easing your state, sleep becomes possible again.

'But they don't send me back to sleep!' I hear you say, and there lies a big problem – most people have used anxiety reduction and relaxation techniques, but have very unhelpful expectations that they should make them go back to sleep. Except, they are designed to reduce your anxiety and relax you and are nothing to do with sleep. How can you focus on that goal if you're too busy thinking about 'sleep, sleep, sleep' all the time? And how on earth are you ever going to sleep if you can't get rid of the anxiety? So these tools must come with acceptance – the overall goal here is to get rid of the overthinking about the day and/or the sleep anxiety gremlins. Reducing anxiety can only really help you sleep if you are working on your sleep baseline and strengthening that sleep muscle of yours.

Things that don't help (even though they're tempting)

- Checking the time. We've seen that glancing at the clock fuels panic and pressure. It shifts your mindset from *rest* to *race against the clock* – and sleep hates a deadline.

- Scrolling your phone. Even if it's just for 'a few minutes', the information and stimulation are like caffeine for your brain. (Plus, the algorithm is designed to keep you awake.)

- Telling yourself the day is ruined. Remember, one bad night doesn't equal a bad day. You've survived worse.

Your body is adaptable – and you don't need perfect sleep to function.

- Overthinking your sleep strategy. 'Should I get up? Try a different technique? Move rooms?' If you're layering fourteen strategies on top of each other, pause. Breathe. Choose one simple action and let go of the rest. (You might want to decide on this the night before so you're not left in decision paralysis in the middle of the night.) Less really is more.

Overthinking Without the Anxiety

Sometimes, the racing mind and repetitive songs playing out in your head don't feel like sleep anxiety, they are just there, at the wrong times, and can even be related to having a really good day. If this happens to you once in a while, I say just ride the wave, distract yourself and follow the advice in this book to stop it worrying you. If it's super regular, then allowing your brain some time for processing before you intend to sleep can be very helpful. Yes, your sleep has stages that usually take care of all that mental processing, but our data consumption during the day through the speedy rise in technology has surpassed our capacity to evolve quickly enough to deal with it. Essentially, we are still mentally processing our lives much the same way as we did when there was no Netflix and we spent hours by the fire instead and participating in our cave-people responsibilities.

So, how to deal with this? Give your brain an opportunity each day before the evening – and ideally several times during the day – to stop, reflect, zone out, stare off into space or journal. Letting thoughts run freely, or reflecting on your day in a more structured way, gives your brain a chance to process what's going on and leaves you less 'buzzy' at night. You're not trying to force anything – just making space. And, as ever, all of this works far better if your sleep baseline is strong and you follow the habit with some consistency.

One simple way to give your brain a chance to offload before bed is to try writing down three things you're grateful for, two things you learned today and one thing you're looking forward to tomorrow. It's a small habit that can help clear mental clutter while reinforcing a positive mindset. Over time, your brain will start to recognize that this is its daily opportunity to process and reflect, so it doesn't need to hijack your thoughts later when you're trying to sleep.

Here's the truth: the gremlins will visit again. They always do. But the next time they show up, you'll be ready. You'll remind yourself that sleep isn't something you control minute by minute – it's a long-term relationship. You'll embrace the fact that your body is resilient, that one bad night won't ruin you and that you don't need to fight wakefulness. And as you learn to let go, you'll notice something incredible: the gremlins lose their power over time – you are desensitizing yourself. And when they do, you'll finally feel what it's like to sleep freely – without fear.

Now that we've calmed the sleep anxiety gremlins, or at least taken away their megaphone, the next instinct is often to fix the 'damage'. We tell ourselves that we need to catch up, to make up for bad nights like we're settling a debt.

It's a tempting idea – sleep as a currency, hours in and out, balance restored. But sleep doesn't work like a bank. And trying to treat it like one might be the very thing stopping it from working in your favour... we will explore this in the next chapter.

CHAPTER 6

Sleep Isn't a Bank: Stop Making Deposits

The problem: We've been taught that sleep works like a bank: lose hours, pay them back.
The fix: Chasing lost hours just breaks your rhythm and your sleep ends up worse, not better. Real recovery comes from consistency, not compensation.

Let's start with a reminder of what we learned in Part 1: sleep debt is not the simple 'eye-for-an-eye' repayment system we've been led to believe. If you lose sleep, your body doesn't demand every lost hour back. Instead, it's far more efficient – it prioritizes the stages of sleep that you need most and recalibrates itself naturally. This selective rebound is why you can have a rough week of short nights and bounce back with just one or two nights of slightly longer (possibly, but not always guaranteed), higher-quality sleep.

If you lose sleep, your body doesn't demand every lost hour back. Instead, it's far more efficient – it prioritizes the stages of sleep that you need most and recalibrates itself naturally.

In this chapter, we'll dig deeper into how the body adapts to sleep loss and dispel some of the myths and misunderstandings that keep us trapped in cycles of bad sleep, anxiety and frustration. Trying to 'make up' lost hours with erratic sleep patterns throws off your circadian rhythm, and that makes recovery harder. It's not the lost hours that ruin our sleep – it's the way we try to repay them.

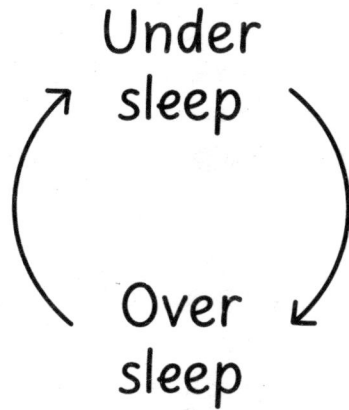

Sleep debt myths aren't just frustrating – they actively make your sleep worse. We touched on our most misunderstood sleep behaviours like lying in, napping and spending more time in bed earlier in the book, but, here, we're going deeper. Because once you understand how damaging the 'sleep as a bank' mindset can be, you'll start to see why lie-ins, for example, although tempting, often make things worse in the long run. These behaviours, when used frequently, are the most common ways people accidentally break their sleep rhythm – and are some of the hardest habits to rethink.

Lie-Ins: The Family Weekend Trap

It's Saturday morning. You've had a long week juggling work, the kids' activities and school runs, and now it's your chance to sleep in while your partner handles breakfast. You tell yourself you're 'catching up', but, by Sunday night, you're lying awake, unable to fall asleep. The next morning, the 6 a.m. alarm feels brutal, and the cycle starts all over again. This is a classic case of 'social jet lag', where weekend lie-ins throw off your circadian rhythm. It's like shifting your internal clock two hours ahead every Friday night and then forcing it back on Monday morning – like the clock change, except you're putting yourself through it over and over again. And it doesn't just apply to adults – kids experience it too. When families let children stay up late or sleep in on weekends, their school-week schedules suffer, making weekday mornings harder for everyone.

Take Sarah and Matt, parents of two kids under ten. Their oldest, Jack, loves staying up late on Friday nights to play video games, and their youngest, Lily, wakes them up at 5.30 a.m. regardless. By Sunday night, Jack struggles to fall asleep, Sarah feels groggy from a lie-in and Matt is irritable from trying to catch a nap that didn't help. When the family stuck to the same wake-up time

– even on weekends – things began to improve. And, in Lily's case (because no one wanted to start at 5.30 a.m.!), she wasn't forced to 'try' to stay sleeping, she was simply encouraged to keep her activities similar to those she did before bed (reading, curtains still shut, little light not big light on) until their family get-up time, and Sarah and Matt stopped relying on naps and coffee to get through the week. And because the whole family were more in sync, which meant that their behaviours and activities during the day were happening in sync, even Lily started to stay asleep until the family get-up time.

It didn't work perfectly every weekend – nothing ever does – but most of the time, the shift helped. And that's the point: not perfection, just progress. I appreciate that this is quite different to what a lot of families do right now and so can seem very unrelatable at first, and it's easy to think, 'That won't work for us,' but you would be surprised that the families I've worked with who chose to stick to it for a few weeks as consistently as they could (even if it wasn't perfect) saw the same changes.

The Saturday Afternoon Nap Trap

Naps feel innocent – a harmless luxury. But when they're long, late or frequent, they can quietly sabotage your sleep.

Matt, already groggy from trying to lie in, would often sneak in a Saturday afternoon nap 'just to catch up'. It became a habit – forty minutes, then an hour, sometimes more. But instead of helping, it made things worse. By bedtime, he'd feel wide awake, then grumpy and overtired by Sunday evening, starting the week in a fog.

What he hadn't realized was that the naps were disrupting more than just his schedule – they were eroding his ability to fall asleep easily at night and fragmenting his sleep when it did come. He started noticing more middle-of-the-night wake-ups and, even when he thought he'd slept for hours, he'd wake up feeling unrefreshed. The link wasn't obvious at first – naps seemed harmless – but they were quietly draining his sleep drive and delaying that natural evening sleepiness.

Matt replaced his naps with short walks or quiet time with the kids. At first, it felt counter-intuitive – how could less rest help with tiredness? But once his sleep stabilized, he fell asleep more easily and at a more consistent time (most of the time), his night-time awakenings reduced and his mornings felt clearer. He didn't just feel more rested – he felt more *in control*. It turned out that building a stronger, more predictable sleep drive during the day helped fill in the very sleep gaps he was trying to nap his way out of.

Sleep Deprivation Versus Poor Sleep Quality: Are You Truly in Debt?

One of the biggest misconceptions about sleep debt is the assumption that feeling tired automatically means you're sleep-deprived. We circled around this idea in Chapter 2 – that how much sleep you get and how much rest you feel aren't always the same thing. Now, it's time to unpack why that matters, and how to know which one you're really dealing with.

Sometimes, the issue isn't how much sleep you've had – it's the quality of that sleep. For example, a restless night might leave you feeling groggy, but if your body managed to fit in enough deep and REM sleep, you might function surprisingly well. Conversely, you could get a solid block of hours but feel unrefreshed because your sleep quality was poor – fragmented by stress, alcohol or other disruptions.

Sleep deprivation happens when there's a lack of opportunity to sleep. Maybe you stayed up late bingeing a series or you were woken up repeatedly by a teething baby. In these cases, your body wanted to sleep but couldn't because external circumstances got in the way.

This is different from insomnia, for example, where you often do have the opportunity to sleep – you're in bed, it's quiet and you're ready – but sleep just doesn't come. Insomnia is usually caused by disruptions to your sleep mechanisms (sleep drive and circadian rhythm) plus other factors (which we'll discuss in the appendix), not a simple lack of sleep. In fact, when your body has been actively restricted from sleep, you will see the opposite of insomnia – you won't be able to keep your eyes open... which does seem crazy since anyone suffering from insomnia will tell you that the symptoms of insomnia, all the fatigue and side effects – all they make you feel you want to do is recover lost sleep. However, if it were that simple, you would just spend more time in bed and, voila, the problem would be resolved. This isn't the case, though, and hence why sleep duration is often not a metric for understanding how sleep is. Often during the day or night, people describe that 'tired but wired' feeling that comes along with this type of sleep disruption. This isn't about external factors; it's an internal mismatch where your brain and body aren't aligned with sleep drive or circadian rhythms in that moment.

Why does this matter? Because the way we address these two situations is completely different. For sleep deprivation, your body will recover naturally if given the chance (selectively rebounding by increasing certain stages of sleep and some duration). For insomnia, trying to force sleep or 'catch up' only reinforces the underlying anxiety and misalignment that caused the problem in the first place.

Here's where things get tricky: sleep deprivation and insomnia can overlap. You might be sleep-deprived from a crying baby, a demanding job or late-night chores, but when you finally do get the opportunity to sleep, because of a misalignment between your sleep mechanisms, as described above, you find yourself lying awake, unable to switch off. It's a vicious cycle: your body needs sleep, but your mind won't let it happen. So what do you do then? Create more opportunity for sleep – but that doesn't mean forcing an early bedtime. As you'll remember from Chapter 4, going to bed too early can backfire. Instead, go to bed when you genuinely feel sleepy-tired. If that happens to be earlier than usual, great – take advantage of it. But let the feeling lead, not the clock. You also need to maintain that get-up time that we established on page 100. This keeps your sleep baseline strong, aligns with your internal master clock and builds a predictable sleep drive – so your body naturally recovers any sleep debt. Something important to reiterate here: you cannot start with the evening – you have to make sure the get-up time is consistent before listening to what your body wants, otherwise those sleepy-tired feelings in the evening will be all over the place and, before you know it, you're in bed sleeping at 8 p.m., only to be wide awake by 11 p.m.

How do I know when I'm sleepy-tired?

This is a very good question. There is a huge difference between being fatigue tired – aching, sore eyes, mental fog, can't concentrate, pain, feeling like you need to 'rest' and many other things – and sleepy-tired: that feeling where you just cannot keep your eyes open. That's it. It's the only definition – you are fighting to literally keep yourself awake. Sometimes, people are so wedded to their bedtimes that they never experience this; these are the people who can end up lying in bed awake for hours. If this sounds like you, don't panic – it takes practice and a bit of trial and error to figure this one out. You can do it, even if it means a few late nights to start with.

This also usually brings up further issues with daytime sleepiness and/or fatigue. Feeling fatigue during the day often means you need to take some type of rest (maybe it's getting out of your office environment or just resting your body on the sofa) – but not a nap rest. As we've seen, forcing yourself to take a nap can lead to complications with your sleep. Sometimes, if the environment is right and you had a rough night, a nap might work. But even that can have consequences over time – fragmenting your sleep further and training your brain to feel sleepy at the wrong times during the day. That's not to say the odd nap is always going to be bad for you, but hopefully by now you're learning that consistency in your behaviours leads to patterns, good and bad.

A little note here about sleep disorders: if you find you can't get through the day without napping just to 'cope' very regularly, check out the appendix (page 273) as this can be a sign of a sleep disorder.

When it comes to knowing whether you're sleep-deprived, this is where perception complicates things again. As mentioned, we are notoriously bad at judging how much we've actually slept. Add in sleep trackers, which can misreport sleep stages, and you've got a recipe for unnecessary worry. People often become fixated on 'catching up' based on tracker data or subjective feelings, and both could be wrong or simply encourage you into the wrong behaviours.

Sarah, the mum from earlier, found herself stuck in another common trap: the sleep debt loop. After several rough nights with her toddler Lily – and 'proof' from her sleep tracker that her hours were too low – she started going to bed an hour early to 'catch up'. But instead of drifting off, she'd lie there wide awake, trapped in that 'tired but wired' state. On the rare occasions Lily slept in, Sarah would do the same – only to wake groggy, heavy-headed and no more refreshed.

What she didn't realize was that her early bedtimes and occasional lie-ins were quietly breaking her rhythm. Her sleep became patchy and unpredictable. Even on nights when she technically got more sleep, she didn't feel better. It wasn't until she stopped trying to force recovery and instead waited until she felt genuinely sleepy – while sticking to a regular get-up time – that her sleep began to settle. That extra hour in the evening turned into a wind-down period instead of a battleground.

And maybe most important of all: she stopped

monitoring her sleep through her tracker, which helped her to start trusting rest over chasing sleep. Just resting on the sofa, reading or staring into space became enough. And when sleep did come, it came more easily. She no longer felt like she was constantly falling behind.

The three sleep situations and what to do in each

1. Sleep deprivation (you didn't get enough sleep, but your body can sleep):

Example: You were up with the baby, travelling, working really late or binge-watching TV.

Your body wants sleep and will take it when it gets the chance.

What to do:

- Don't go to bed early unless you genuinely feel sleepy-tired (can't keep your eyes open). This will likely be earlier if you are genuinely sleep-deprived – don't worry if it's not!

- Stick to your usual get-up time to avoid throwing off your rhythm.

- Over the next night or two, your body will naturally rebalance if it needs to, no special effort needed.

You're tired because you missed sleep. The fix is consistency, not overcompensation.

2. Insomnia (you're in bed, you want to sleep – but can't):

Example: You're lying awake at 2 a.m., feeling tired but wired. There's no external reason, your brain just won't switch off. This is about misalignment, not sleep loss.

What to do:

- Do not nap or lie in the next day, it keeps the misalignment going.
- Only go to bed when you feel genuinely sleepy-tired, even if it's late.
- Keep your get-up time consistent to rebuild sleep drive and rhythm.
- Focus on low-pressure rest (reading, sitting on the sofa) to reduce sleep anxiety.

You're not lacking sleep time, you're lacking the conditions for sleep to kick in. The fix is rhythm, not sleep quantity.

3. Mixed state (you were sleep-deprived, now you're wired and can't recover):

Example: After a rough week with broken sleep, you finally have a quiet night, but now you still can't fall asleep. Your sleep systems are out of sync: high need, low ability.

What to do:

- Keep a firm get-up time to re-anchor your rhythm.
- At night, wait until you feel that unmistakable sleepy-tired feeling.

- Use the evening to relax without trying to force sleep (wind down instead of lie down).
- Avoid lie-ins and naps, even if you're tempted, let the rhythm rebuild.

You're stuck in between. The fix is routine, patience and pressure-free evenings.

Notice how there is not much difference between these approaches, and yet they allow you enough flexibility to recover in the way your body really needs to at the time, rather than what we have traditionally done, which leads to more frustration and anxiety, but not the sleep you are after!

Sleep debt doesn't work in the way we think it does. It's not about repaying hours – it's about supporting your body's natural recovery systems with consistency and care. Whether you're juggling family life, work stress or both, remember: the key to better sleep isn't 'catching up' – it's letting go of perfection, trusting your body and focusing on the bigger picture.

It's time to move from the most common and misunderstood sleep behaviours to the sleep tools we are told we cannot live without. From sleep trackers to supplements, weighted blankets to sprays, the next chapter is your ultimate guide to the gadgets we're told we need – and what the evidence really says about them.

CHAPTER 7

The Sleep Tools Trap: When Help Stops Helping

The problem: We're obsessing over sleep gadgets and supplements that promise big results but deliver little – and often make sleep anxiety worse.

The fix: Focus on what actually works: a strong sleep baseline, consistent routines and realistic expectations. Tools can help if used wisely, but they're never the fix on their own.

In today's world, sleep is often presented as a problem that can be solved with the right quick-fix tool. The market is flooded with trackers, sprays, vitamins, blankets, noise machines and apps – each promising to unlock the secret to a perfect night's rest. But here's the truth: these tools are often a distraction, offering marginal improvements at best. Many of us are drawn to the idea of fine-tuning our bodies for those 1–2 per cent gains, but that only works if you've already addressed the fundamentals of sleep first. The real solution isn't in a gadget or pill – it's in understanding and nurturing the sleep mechanisms your body already has. Also, all these sleep tools come with a hidden cost if we're not careful: they distract us from the real solutions, reinforce unhealthy beliefs and keep us locked in cycles of anxiety. This is not me pooh-poohing a whole industry; I actually think that some of the gadgets could be very useful and beneficial if only they were marketed slightly differently, and we held some accountability for what we are creating. But unfortunately, the most profitable way of selling them is just slapping 'sleep aid' on it, and this is where the problem begins. What does that even mean?

I thought long and hard about writing this chapter because I don't want to confuse you further or indeed dictate what suits you in your life – you do you, my friend, that's most important. What I would like to do is cut through the noise and help you understand the influence of certain things. So that when you choose what you want to do, you're not doing it because you're worried about the consequences of not doing it, and that it actually brings you consistent support/joy/whatever it is you're after.

Why We're Obsessed with Sleep Tools

Sleep is one of the few biological processes we can't consciously control, and that lack of control is unsettling – especially when we finally realize how important it is for our health. The marketplace has stepped in, offering products that promise to give us control and reassurance, even though the actual impact is often negligible. It's no coincidence that the global sleep aids market was valued at over $70 billion in 2024 – and it's still growing. Your body already knows how to sleep. It's our habits, beliefs and anxieties that interfere. And yet, we reach for tools that can, at best, treat the symptoms while ignoring the root cause, and often increase our anxieties around sleep, not liberate us from them. So, let's go through a selection and then, at the end of the chapter, I'll give you a helpful tool to navigate it all more effectively.

It's not just that these gadgets are marketed as fixes for our sleep – it's that we're told we need them to function in a society where 'better' sleep means 'more productive' lives. The sleep industry has become a multi-billion-dollar machine, and it's easy to see how we, as consumers, are influenced by its promises of quick fixes. The reality is, sleep isn't a commodity you can buy in a pill or a device. And the more we're sold on the idea of 'hacks' and 'perfect sleep', the further we move away from understanding the deep, real work that goes into creating a healthy sleep foundation.

First, let's look at one of the most popular sleep tools: sleep trackers. From wristbands to rings to necklaces, these gadgets promise to provide insights into your sleep patterns, giving you the illusion of control. But, as with most sleep tools, there's more to the story than meets the eye.

Sleep Trackers: The Double-Edged Glow of the Wristband/Ring/Necklace

Sleek, tech-savvy and whispering promises of better sleep with the power of 'data', they're everywhere – from your smartwatch to that wearable ring your co-worker swears by. And who wouldn't want to know their sleep score, right? It feels empowering to quantify the mysterious hours you spend unconscious. But here's the truth about sleep trackers: they might be doing more harm than good for many of us. Yes, they look cool and seem insightful, but beneath the glossy interface, they're often inaccurate, misleading and even anxiety-inducing. Let's break down the good, the bad and the downright confusing reality of sleep trackers.

The appeal of sleep trackers

For some, the data from a sleep tracker can be a helpful nudge to improve habits, like sticking to a consistent get-up time or avoiding late-night scrolling. Awareness is powerful, and sleep trackers certainly provide that. If you're using a tracker for big-picture insights rather than nightly micromanagement, they can be helpful. Over time, you might notice patterns like worse sleep on nights when you drink or better sleep when you exercise. Trends can guide smarter decisions, as long as you don't read them as gospel (you can put a good night's sleep and exercise together, but it doesn't mean that will work every time, as this entire book explains). If you feel the correlational data shows you cause and effect, it can lead to disappointment when your sleep doesn't reach your expectations.

Most consumer-grade sleep trackers use a combination of motion sensors (actigraphy) and heart rate monitoring to infer sleep stages. But here's the catch: they're not measuring your actual sleep. Unlike polysomnography (the gold standard used in sleep clinics), which tracks brainwaves, sleep trackers rely on algorithms to guess if you're asleep, awake or in a specific sleep stage. Have you ever binged a Netflix series while lying still and later saw your tracker credit you with an hour of 'light sleep'? Trackers are great at detecting movement, but terrible at understanding why you're not moving. Many trackers claim to provide data on REM, light sleep and deep sleep. But studies show they're less than 50 per cent accurate at identifying these stages compared to polysomnography. So, when your app proudly tells you that you had 17 per cent REM sleep, take it with a very large pinch of salt.

A sleep tracker doesn't know you had an argument with your partner before bed, drank three espressos at 9 p.m. or are recovering from a cold. Sleep is highly individual, and no algorithm can capture the nuances of why you slept poorly one night and better the next (not yet anyway). Also, bear in mind what we discussed in Chapter 1 about sleep stages: the fact that you only spent around 20 per cent of your time in REM is normal and you can't really increase it on a regular basis in a healthy way. But without that vital bit of information, it's easy to think it should be higher.

For example, a study published in *Sleep Health* found that sleep trackers often overestimate total sleep time and underestimate how often you wake up during the night, and have poor detection of accurate sleep stages. This means that while trackers might look like they're giving you insight, they're often guessing – and sometimes guessing wrong. This can lead to unnecessary worry and misplaced solutions. It's crucial to understand that your sleep isn't defined by a score or a number, but by how you feel during the day. Furthermore, when we manipulate the tracker results in studies to show poor sleep – even when it's been good – the health outcomes are much the same as someone who did indeed sleep poorly. This is a crucial finding because it shows how influential these devices can be. Even when the data is false, it can have the same negative effects on your mental state as actual poor sleep. In other words, the sleep tracker doesn't just track your sleep – it can track your anxiety too.

The problem is, even if they are 100 per cent accurate, and I'm sure one day they will be, they are still encouraging you to micromanage sleep on a nightly basis, by providing you with data with not much context. The art of sleep ebbing and flowing and adjusting as needed according to the constant changes in our environment and our biology is completely ignored. The unintended result can instead be orthosomnia, when you become so obsessed with achieving the 'perfect' sleep score that it actually makes your sleep worse. Yes, the very device designed to help you sleep better might be keeping you awake. Expectations, disappointment, fear... it's a vicious cycle.

Mei, a thirty-four-year-old teacher, came to me after months of poor sleep. She wasn't sure why her sleep was deteriorating but kept pointing to her tracker: 'It says I'm not getting enough REM sleep. That must be why I'm so tired.' I get this story a lot. But when I looked at her sleep tracker and her REM cycles (if we are indeed going to believe in what it was showing us), I actually saw a pretty healthy REM distribution over a week. Mei was encouraged to think that the percentage of REM she was getting was not enough. This was sending her down strange paths when it came to trying to fix her 'REM problem'. She would look for aids that specifically talked about consistently increasing REM, even though that's not really possible. Mei's sleep really was in need of improving, especially because since this entire debacle began, her healthy sleep behaviours had actually declined: she started to sleep in and go to bed early because she was feeling exhausted, cancelling daytime activities with friends and not exercising; she had completely moved away from her healthy sleep–wake pattern. After ditching the tracker and focusing on a consistent get-up time and light exposure, and helping her deal with those pesky sleep anxiety gremlins in the short term, she slept better within weeks.

Mei realized that the tracker had become a mirror to her anxiety about sleep. Every night, she was letting her tracker dictate whether or not she was 'worthy' of a good night's sleep. The moment she disconnected from that anxiety and started focusing on her routine, her true restfulness returned.

A 2017 study in *Journal of Clinical Sleep Medicine* documented cases of orthosomnia caused by sleep trackers. Participants became hyper-focused on their data, which heightened their anxiety and perpetuated sleep problems.

When your sleep tracker gives you a poor score, it's easy to believe you slept badly, even if you woke up feeling fine. This can lead to a self-fulfilling prophecy: you start to worry about your sleep, which increases anxiety, which worsens your sleep. Imagine waking up refreshed, only to see your tracker say you got four hours of sleep. Now you feel tired, even though you didn't before. That's the psychological power of suggestion. Trackers encourage us to micromanage something we're better off leaving alone. Sleep is a natural process, and obsessing over metrics can distract from what actually matters: how you feel during the day and whether you're mostly maintaining healthy sleep habits. The more you rely on external tools, the less you trust your body to regulate sleep on its own. This reliance can lead to a dependency that's hard to break, especially when you're convinced the tracker knows better than you.

Luis, a forty-year-old lawyer, came to me convinced he had insomnia because his tracker consistently showed poor sleep efficiency. But Luis wasn't struggling to fall asleep or stay asleep – his tracker was simply misreading his midnight trips to the bathroom as extended wake periods. Once we debunked the tracker's data and worked on his confidence, his 'insomnia' magically disappeared.

Sleep trackers might not seem harmful, but they can lead to behaviours that actively interfere with sleep, like what Mei was doing. We often overcompensate for perceived poor sleep by changing our routines – going to bed earlier, sleeping in or skipping exercise – all of which disrupt circadian rhythms and sleep drive. Misinterpreting tracker data can lead people to seek medical help when none is needed or, worse, self-prescribe supplements or medications without addressing the real issue (and just wasting money instead).

A smarter way to use sleep trackers

Sleep trackers aren't inherently bad. The key is to use them as a tool for general trends, not a nightly report card. I personally believe they need to be designed entirely differently in order to help you do this (ahem sleep tracker developers!), but, if you're careful, you can use them in a healthier way:

Do:
- Look for patterns over weeks or months rather than obsessing over daily fluctuations.
- Pair tracking with actionable goals, like setting a consistent get-up time or getting more light exposure.
- Ignore the actual numbers and percentages – just use them as a baseline of where you started and do not forget context. If you're on your period or you find yourself quite stressed, then your sleep will be more varied than usual. And this is normal.

Don't:
- Treat the data as gospel – you know more about your sleep than it does. Focus on the feels!
- Use your tracker to micromanage your sleep. Focus on consistency and simple influential habits, not nightly perfection.

- Let poor scores dictate how you feel during the day, or poor sleep for that matter (and we will get to the how in Part 3). Be careful here – even letting a 'good' sleep score dictate how you feel isn't ideal, as this only reinforces how badly you might feel when the score isn't 'good'.

Sleep trackers can be useful, but only if you approach them with the right mindset. They're not medical devices, and they're not a substitute for understanding the fundamentals of sleep. Instead of obsessing over numbers, focus on what you've learned in this book: strengthening your sleep drive, aligning with your circadian rhythm and reducing sleep anxiety. Your body already knows how to sleep – it doesn't need a gadget to tell it how. Trust your instincts, not your tracker, and remember: the best tool for better sleep is you.

The Sleep Supplements Showdown: Hype versus Science

Supplements have become the darlings of the sleep world. Walk into any health store – or scroll through Instagram for five seconds – and you'll be hit with promises of deep, uninterrupted sleep in a bottle, often from health and well-being folk. Magnesium, melatonin, valerian root, CBD oil, 5-HTP, L-theanine... It's an alphabet soup of alleged sleep cures. But do they work?

Your body already knows how to sleep – it doesn't need a gadget to tell it how. Trust your instincts, not your tracker.

And, more importantly, are they actually helping you in the long run? Because it's definitely an added financial burden, that's for sure!

Let's dive into the most popular sleep supplements, their supposed magic, the science behind them (or lack thereof) and why they might not be the harmless helpers they claim to be.

Magnesium: the OG sleep hero?

The claim: Magnesium relaxes your muscles, calms your nerves and helps you drift off like a baby in a hammock. It's often touted as the ultimate sleep enhancer, especially for those with stress or insomnia.

The reality: Magnesium is indeed involved in hundreds of biochemical processes in your body, including ones that affect sleep. But here's the catch: unless you're clinically deficient (which is rare in developed countries, and you need a blood test to quantify this), taking extra magnesium is unlikely to improve your sleep. One review found that magnesium supplements may help older adults with insomnia, but the effects were mild at best – and largely limited to those with a clinical deficiency.

Also, I've seen clients who genuinely did have a clinical magnesium deficiency, diagnosed by an actual doctor, but because they started supplementing after the first few months (if not years) of getting poor sleep, the new broken sleep pattern became ingrained (remember how smart that brain is). So, correcting the original deficiency didn't actually take away the insomnia.

Meet Diego, a stressed-out accountant in his late forties. He came to my clinic clutching a tub of magnesium gummies, convinced they were his 'sleep salvation'. Despite months of popping them like candy, his sleep hadn't improved. We ran tests and found his magnesium levels were fine. Also, he was having other symptoms caused by taking too much magnesium. What Diego really needed was an education on how to improve his sleep baseline with the most influential behaviours. Once he did, his sleep improved – and he then chose to save the £40 a month he used to spend on gummies. He now had evidence there was some influence he could have with far simpler tools, plus his expectations around sleep were managed.

Diego wasn't just frustrated by the gummies – he was frustrated with the idea that sleep was something he had to force with a supplement. His anxiety about sleep became so entwined with the idea that 'he needed something' to get it that he forgot that sleep could be simple, natural and trustworthy. That's what I see time and again: people becoming so reliant on pills or products that they lose sight of their body's own ability to rest. But when Diego took a step back and asked himself, 'What if I don't need a pill? What if it is my habits that need changing instead?', he was able to slowly shift his sleep pattern with simple changes, and that was far more powerful than any supplement.

You see, even if magnesium doesn't work, people often feel they need it to sleep. This creates a dependency that undermines their confidence in their body's natural ability to rest. And when you inevitably forget your magnesium on holiday? Cue the anxiety gremlins. Also, like most things, including most supplements, everything in moderation. People don't realize that too much magnesium is not good – it's not a simple harmless placebo at best. It can cause havoc with certain medications, have side effects like digestive issues, muscle issues or even kidney strain, to name but a few. So, if you want to use magnesium, please do, but promise me you will speak to your medical practitioner first – especially if you have other chronic conditions and/or are taking medication.

Melatonin: the hormone everyone thinks they need

The claim: Melatonin, the 'sleep hormone', regulates your body clock. Taking it as a supplement should magically reset your sleep and fix jet lag, insomnia or any late-night Netflix binges.

The reality: Melatonin can work, but only in very specific situations. And, even then, it rarely does more than what you could achieve naturally by strengthening your sleep baseline. It's most effective for:

- 🕐 Jet lag – when your body clock needs a nudge to align with a new time zone. (Though I don't take it for jet lag because I know my sleep will adjust, and I can help it naturally by looking after the things I have control over – like getting up, getting light and eating, all when the locals do!)
- 🕐 Circadian sleep problems such as delayed sleep phase disorder. This is a rare genetic condition where your body clock is naturally out of sync. Often this is supplemented with bright light exposure and taking care of your sleep baseline. On its own, or used at the wrong times, melatonin can actually make this condition worse.

For everyone else? Studies show melatonin has minimal impact. A meta-analysis found that melatonin improved sleep onset by an average of seven minutes. Seven! That's barely enough time to scroll through TikTok once. On this note, take care when studies show these marginal improvements in sleep onset efficiency and sleep duration – if you have a chronic sleep problem that is affecting your life significantly, it is not an extra five minutes of sleep you need. You need an overhaul of your sleep system where the timing, quality and duration are taken into consideration.

Melatonin doesn't make you sleep – it tells your body it's bedtime. If your circadian rhythm is already aligned (thanks to Chapter 4), popping melatonin is like sending a calendar invite for a meeting that's already happening. Sometimes it can feel like it is doing something – but very briefly. The problem is, if you felt it sort of did something at some point, you might be desperate enough to keep using it 'just in case'.

And yes, melatonin can also have side effects. The most common evidence-based side effects of melatonin are daytime drowsiness, vivid dreams or nightmares, dizziness, headaches and gastrointestinal discomfort. While long-term impact is less clear at this point (because of the lack of studies), I am starting to see in clinic an increase in people using it in the long term, without it resolving their sleep issues, and causing what seems to be a psychological dependency, which only adds a layer of complication when treating the original sleep condition.

Valerian root: the 'natural' remedy

The claim: Valerian root is a centuries-old herbal remedy that calms the mind and induces sleep. Think of it as nature's sedative.

The reality: Valerian root has shown some promise in reducing anxiety and improving sleep latency (time to fall asleep) in certain studies, but the effects are modest. A review in *Sleep Medicine Reviews* found valerian to be 'possibly effective', but noted that many studies were poorly designed or too small to draw strong conclusions.

Valerian's effects are inconsistent, and side effects like headaches and dizziness are common. Plus, 'natural' doesn't mean 'harmless'. Herbal supplements can interact with medications, so taking valerian without consulting a doctor is risky.

Ali, a friend and teacher in their fifties, swore by valerian tea before bed: 'It has to be working – it smells so awful though!' they joked. But when I enquired a little deeper, their consistent morning routine and cut off from the day where they actively enjoyed their evening without those usual daytime activities was likely doing more for their sleep than the tea itself. We replaced valerian with a cup of chamomile (and, before you ask, the sleep evidence for chamomile is mild at its very best) and, guess what? They slept just as well – without the side effects.

CBD oil: the trendy newcomer

The claim: CBD (cannabidiol) is touted to reduce anxiety, relax the body and promote deeper sleep – all without the psychoactive effects of THC (tetrahydrocannabinol – the bit that produces 'the high').

The reality: The enthusiasm surrounding CBD often surpasses the current scientific evidence. While some studies suggest potential benefits, their methodologies frequently lack robustness. For instance, one systematic review highlighted that many studies reporting improvements in insomnia symptoms had significant limitations, including small sample sizes and non-validated subjective measures. Also, I personally roll my eyes when studies show 'improvement in insomnia symptoms' – notice how they don't say 'abolition' of insomnia, or measure how subjects feel overall about their insomnia now they are taking CBD oil. Still got sleep anxiety? Check. Still have seriously broken sleep that impacts your life significantly even though it's marginally improved? Check. Moreover, the long-term effects and safety of CBD use remain under-researched, necessitating more rigorous, large-scale and controlled trials to draw definitive conclusions.

CBD products are largely unregulated, meaning quality and dosage can vary wildly. Plus, they're expensive. Why spend £60 on a bottle of CBD oil when you could invest in a simple better morning routine? And why would you use it to try to 'treat' your decades-old debilitating sleep disorder insomnia if we actually have an extremely evidence-based solution to absolutely get rid of your insomnia? (And we will talk about this more in the appendix – see page 273.)

5-HTP and L-theanine: the 'mood boosters'

The claim: 5-HTP (a precursor to serotonin) and L-theanine (an amino acid found in tea) promote relaxation and improve sleep quality.

The reality: While 5-HTP may boost serotonin, its effects on sleep are minimal. It's also not recommended for long-term use due to potential side effects, including gastrointestinal issues and interactions with antidepressants.

L-theanine can promote relaxation and reduce stress, making it a 'nice' pre-bedtime tea ingredient. But its direct impact on sleep is minimal.

The danger of sleep supplement dependency

Every time you pop a supplement, you're telling your brain, 'I can't sleep without this.' Over time, this creates a psychological dependency, where the mere thought of running out of pills triggers panic. They also distract from the real solutions: understanding sleep and managing expectations/sleep anxiety, improving your sleep baseline and, if needed, actual chronic sleep disorder medical intervention, which exists by the way – it's not all just Instagram hacks! Supplements for sleep are like fixing a leaky roof by repainting the ceilings – it might look better, but the problem remains.

The Sleep Tools: Noises, Sprays, Stories and Everything Else You've Been Sold

Priya and Scott have three kids. Their household looks like a sleep tech showroom: sound machines, lavender diffusers and matching weighted blankets for everyone. But despite all the 'tools', Priya still lies awake worrying about whether they 'missed something'. When they focused instead on consistent routines for the kids (and themselves) and improving their sleep baseline, they realized they didn't need all the gadgets and most of them ended up on eBay.

Let's dive into the wonderfully cluttered world of sleep tools to hopefully help you make your decisions. These tools often have cult followings, glowing testimonials and clever marketing campaigns. But how much do they really help? Are they harmless comforts or traps for over-reliance? Spoiler: the answer depends on how – and why – you use them.

Weighted blankets: cosy or overrated?

Weighted blankets are the warm, heavy hug you didn't know you needed – until everyone on social media told you they were life-changing. These blankets are marketed as anxiety-reducing and sleep-promoting, and there's some science to show that they can indeed have a subjective, positive effect on some people (those with anxiety-related psychiatric disorders), but are they really the answer to your sleep woes?

The relaxation benefits might help you feel better, but they don't directly address the mechanics of sleep (circadian rhythm, sleep drive, and so on). If your sleep problems are deeply rooted, a weighted blanket won't solve them.

It's interesting because when people realize this, instead of stopping using the weighted blanket, because there is a perception that it works 'sometimes' (and that's more likely because your sleep baseline that day was a bit better!), they get that dependency risk. If you start believing you can't sleep without your weighted blanket, you're setting yourself up for trouble. What happens when you travel or forget it on a trip? When it comes to just using a weighted blanket with an expectation that it might help you relax and not to *make* you sleep, that is a much more reasonable expectation. Of course, some people find the weight suffocating or too warm, especially in hotter climates. So, they're not for everyone.

The verdict: Weighted blankets can be a nice addition to your relaxation routine, if they help you feel a little calmer. But they're not a fix for sleep problems. Have the right expectations.

Noise machines: white, pink, brown...

Whether it's white, pink or brown noise, the idea is to mask disruptive sounds and create a consistent auditory environment that is comfortable. But how much do they help?

White noise is a mix of all sound frequencies, creating a consistent hum. It is popular for blocking out environmental noise (like traffic or snoring, and some people will use it for tinnitus). Studies show that white noise can help people fall asleep faster by masking sudden disruptions. A study in the *Journal of Caring Sciences* found that white noise improved sleep in patients surrounded by constant noise in a coronary care unit. (Note this is not the environment most of us find ourselves in when we go to sleep at night.)

Pink noise emphasizes lower frequencies and is less harsh than white noise. A study in *Frontiers in Human Neuroscience* found that pink noise enhanced slow-wave sleep and memory in older adults. Brown noise focuses on even lower frequencies, creating a deeper, softer sound. It's less studied but might be preferred by people who find white noise too harsh.

The verdict: If you have to sleep in an inconsistently noisy environment that is genuinely breaking your sleep, you may find this tool helpful, but you will need to be consistent with your approach to get used to the noise. However, be mindful of hypersensitivity and other phenomena we start to notice when sleep becomes poor – it could be that your sleep baseline is just very weak and a little bit of work on that makes your sleep system a bit more robust, making you less susceptible to sound (as your RAS helps filter out sounds). Just like weighted blankets, let's not forget that relying on a noise machine can make you feel lost without it.

Sleep sprays: aromatherapy hype?

Lavender pillow sprays are everywhere, promising to lull you to sleep with their calming scents. Aromatherapy is a multi-billion-dollar industry, and sleep sprays are one of its shining stars, using lavender and other scents like chamomile. Look hard enough and you will find studies showing it has some calming effects, and squint even harder and there will be some studies showing it improves sleep. But, just like any study I mention in this book, measuring sleep is often done on human perception or simply measuring one or two factors like duration and sleep onset, which doesn't really tell us much on its own. In this case, what I want to know is how many of the subjects had a strong sleep baseline to start with? How do we measure that?

The verdict: In reality and in clinic, the only time I send someone off to light a candle or make their pillow smell nice is if it makes them happy and there is a positive, psychological association with no fear or worry over what happens if there is no nice smell. Because, ultimately, it's better to be happy most of the time than not!

Sleep stories: adult bedtime tales

Apps like Calm and Headspace have turned bedtime stories into a booming trend for adults. The idea is to distract your brain with soothing narratives, lulling you to sleep. And they absolutely can interrupt racing thoughts and shift your focus to something calming. They can be a great way to unwind and make that transition from work and day, to relax and evening. But that's just it – this should be the expectation, not that they will fix all your sleep issues.

Interestingly, when I do corporate work, most companies employing me have these apps for their employees to use, almost like a tick-box exercise – 'sleep well-being has been covered for all staff'. But when I delve a little deeper, it turns out the sleep problems remain, and all the questions and concerns of the staff are the same as those who don't have these apps in their corporate packages (and hence the usage remains high!). The tick-box exercise should be in relaxation and anxiety reduction with no expectation that they will help with sleep, because the majority of people who consume that message have already got a weak or broken sleep system that requires far more influential practices. And therein lies the issue with a lot of sleep hacks – if your sleep is good, you have a strong sleep baseline and it serves you, how many of you are looking to sleep tools/hacks and solutions? You're just not. In actual fact, the research would be a lot stronger for at least the anxiety reduction and reduction in 'brain chatter' techniques if the people using them were already working from a strong sleep baseline, and were indeed just looking for that 1–2 per cent improvement and enjoyment from sleep. But the reality is that most of us are just not that. It's that sleep marketing again, making you think it's more than it is – slap 'sleep aid' on the ad and you will sell more.

The verdict: Mindfulness and sleep story apps can be helpful wind-down tools, but they're not a fix for broken sleep. Use them to relax, not to repair. The real work starts with rebuilding your sleep baseline.

Earplugs and eye masks

In noisy or bright environments, earplugs and eye masks can be real game changers, especially when travelling. They help block out distractions, creating a more peaceful sleep environment when you can't control the surroundings. However, if you have the opportunity to adjust your environment – like installing blackout curtains or lowering the noise levels – you might find that earplugs and eye masks become less necessary over time. Also do test them before you become too dedicated to them – again, I've seen people with this hot list of non-negotiables for sleep that didn't even come about because there was, for example, a noise or light issue – they had just simply been told that using them would make their sleep better.

The verdict: They're useful in the short term, but you may find that, with the right environmental changes, you don't need them as much.

Bedclothes

There's no shortage of advice on the 'best' fabrics for sleepwear or bedding, with claims that certain materials guarantee better sleep. The truth is, what matters most is comfort. Whether you prefer cotton sheets, silk pyjamas or just sleeping naked, it's about finding what makes you feel most comfortable. We are all so different and it's good that the choice exists, but stick to your own needs here.

The verdict: The latest trends can be tempting, but they're less important than simply making sure your body is at ease and that you're not too hot or too cold. Focus on comfort, not the latest sleepwear fad.

Herbal teas and warm milk

When it comes to old-school remedies, like a warm glass of milk or a soothing herbal tea before bed, you might wonder if there's more to it than just a nice ritual. While certain herbs, such as chamomile, are thought to have mild calming effects, the real benefit of these rituals often lies in the sense of relaxation they provide. It's the act of slowing down and creating a peaceful pre-sleep environment that plays a bigger role than the beverage itself.

The verdict: Whether it's warm milk, herbal tea or another (non-alcoholic!) drink, if it helps signal to your brain that it's time to wind down, it can become a comforting routine. Remember, though, if you don't have that strong sleep baseline or you're relying on these little rituals to make your sleep magically come, it won't.

Brain stimulation devices: high-tech hype

Let's talk about brain stimulation devices, the latest shiny addition to the sleep tools line-up. Brands are promising to revolutionize your sleep with gentle electrical currents, vibrations or auditory cues designed to affect your brain activity. These devices aim to influence the brain's natural rhythms, particularly during sleep. Here's how they typically work:

- Electrical stimulation. Some devices use transcranial electrical stimulation (tES) to send tiny electrical currents through your scalp. These currents are designed to sync with your brainwaves and enhance specific sleep stages, like slow-wave sleep (deep sleep).
- Auditory cues. Other devices play subtle sounds, such as pink noise, timed to specific phases of your sleep cycle. These sounds aim to deepen sleep stages like REM or slow-wave sleep.
- Vibrational feedback. Some products provide gentle vibrations that claim to help relax the nervous system and promote falling asleep faster.

They sound futuristic – and, honestly, kind of cool. But do they work? And more importantly, do you need them?

A small but widely cited study found that transcranial direct current stimulation during sleep enhanced slow-wave activity and improved memory consolidation in participants. However, this was a tightly controlled, short-term lab experiment – not your typical sleepless Tuesday night at home. Another study in *Frontiers in Human Neuroscience* showed that timed auditory stimulation (like pink noise) could increase slow-wave activity during sleep in some participants. But again, these studies are small and often focus on very specific populations, like older adults with mild cognitive impairment. Results from real-world applications are often not significant and subjective. Some say the device enhances their feelings of restfulness; for others, they're just an expensive placebo.

Meet Mal, a forty-one-year-old software engineer who came to me not being able to get to sleep too well and then just having very light sleep all night. He'd tried everything: melatonin, magnesium, sleep sprays and, most recently, a high-tech brain stimulation headband that cost him £600. Mal was obsessed with the data his headband provided – time in slow-wave sleep, REM percentages, 'sleep quality' scores – and used them to micromanage his nights. The headband didn't address Mal's core issues. Instead, it reinforced his belief that his sleep was fundamentally flawed and that he needed external tools to fix it. Fortunately or unfortunately for Mal, the solution was far less exciting, low-tech and, well, probably a bit boring in comparison: building his sleep baseline, managing his expectations around sleep and, of course, getting rid of the pesky sleep anxiety gremlins.

Often, these kind of tools will be used and impressed on pro athletes, and then that's used in marketing – but let's be real here: those athletes have sleep experts who have already taken them through all the steps to really improve their sleep, and this is the cherry on top because they need all the marginal gains they can get when it comes to a very high standard of performance. Most of us are not living on that playing field (but kudos to you if you are). Currently, these tools are pretty expensive – so it's even more important that you really think about what it is you need before you embark on this tech-heavy avenue. Let's not forget these important themes:

- The 'quick fix' illusion. These devices promise to 'hack' your sleep, making you believe you can bypass consistent, boring (but effective) habits like a regular get-up time or morning light exposure. Spoiler: you can't.
- The validation trap. Using one of these devices can make you hyper-focus on sleep metrics, like 'increasing slow-wave sleep by 10 per cent', even if that metric has no tangible impact on how you feel the next day.
- Anxiety amplifier. If the device doesn't work – or stops working – you might feel even more anxious about your sleep, reinforcing the idea that your sleep is 'broken' and can only be fixed by external interventions.

The verdict: If you have done the work – you take care of your sleep and it serves you well – and you are just reaching for the additional titbits (the sleep athletes' 1–2 per cent!) because you genuinely enjoy pushing health boundaries and experimenting and you have the time and money to do so, then I can imagine this would be something interesting to try. Especially if you love your tech! Just don't mistake it for a fix if you haven't laid the proper foundations yet.

Alcohol and Sleep

Alcohol may seem like a helpful aid when you're struggling to get to sleep – I see it a lot in insomnia patients. It can initially make you feel drowsy and relaxed, which is appealing after a long day, and might even have you snoozing quickly. However, while it can help you fall asleep quicker, alcohol disrupts the natural stages of sleep, particularly deep sleep and REM sleep, which, as we've seen, are essential for rest and recovery. What often happens is you might wake up feeling groggy, even though you technically slept longer, but it can also make you wake unable to get back to sleep in that second half of the night as the alcohol is metabolized and you need more. Over time, relying on alcohol to help you sleep only worsens the underlying sleep issues and because you become less sensitive to the alcohol, sometimes an alcohol dependency too, as you need more and more to have that sleepy impact.

Food and Sleep

What and when you eat can play a role in your sleep quality. Heavy meals or spicy foods right before bed can lead to discomfort and indigestion, keeping you awake or interrupting your sleep. Spicy foods can increase your body temperature and make it harder for you to feel comfortable enough to sleep soundly. Here's the thing though, we have all had a later night eating and needed a bit of breathing space to digest before we sleep or just find ourselves too wired to sleep. It's not about obsessing over when you eat, but just being mindful that anything that gives you digestive issues or eating late will, of course, disrupt sleep as your body struggles to do both at the same time efficiently. Still enjoy the odd late meal with friends – yes, it will likely impact that night, but it's not the end of the world and social connection is really important for us humans. Too regularly, I see people never enjoying this kind of event for fear of how it will impact sleep – they move slowly away from the things they once loved in the pursuit of sleep perfection, not realizing that it is in this act that sleep can become more broken.

Physical Activity Before Sleep

If you're used to winding down by flopping onto the sofa, consider adding a bit of movement to your evening routine. A gentle post-dinner walk, some light stretching or even intimacy can help relax your body and prepare it for sleep. These activities lower stress and help regulate your body's natural sleep drive, making it easier to wind down. It's not about going for a strenuous workout, but introducing small, calming activities that signal to your body it's time to rest, which, ironically, can be movement.

The best time of day to do rigorous exercise for fitness really does vary from person to person, and I know a lot of people worry that exercising too close to bedtime will ruin their sleep. But here's the thing: exercise is incredibly important for your overall health and your sleep in the long term. So, rather than avoiding it altogether, try a little experiment. Notice how your sleep responds when you work out in the evening versus earlier in the day. If it does seem to interfere with your sleep, you can adjust, but if it doesn't, there's no need to change what's working.

Sleep Hygiene Rules

I hate the term 'sleep hygiene'; it is so confusing. If you've ever googled 'how to sleep better', you've likely been inundated with 'sleep hygiene' tips, or had a list from your doctor or friends and family. The problem is, this 'list' of things we should do has become long and random, with different tips having a different level of influence, and some being completely useless. I think it's outdated and sending the wrong message. After all, who do you know who sleeps just fine and is living by all these rules? And, by the time someone comes to see me with their debilitating long-term sleep issue, they have tried of all them. So, where are we going wrong?

The origins of this phenomenon started when the term was coined in 1977 by American psychiatrist Peter Hauri, a pioneering sleep researcher who specialized in treating insomnia. Hauri introduced the concept as part of non-pharmacological treatments for sleep issues. His goal was to promote behavioural and environmental practices that support better sleep, offering an alternative to sleeping pills. Sounds great to me. And while they sound logical – Cut caffeine! Keep your room cool! Turn off devices! – their effectiveness is often misunderstood. Let's explore whether these rules actually prevent sleep issues.

If you have had recent, specific disruptions, like a new baby, a stressful job or travel, but otherwise your sleep is usually fine, it can be useful to use 'sleep hygiene' as a checklist (not rules!) for things that might have been altered because of these changes. That means if you look down the list and decide that you have, indeed, gone from two to ten cups of coffee a day to help you cope with the new baby, you may find that a reduction in caffeine will have a significant impact on your sleep. But let's be clear here: if your caffeine consumption hasn't changed and you are fumbling around looking for solutions for a broken sleep issue, reducing caffeine isn't it. Most people I treat now have completely come off caffeine (to no effect on their actual sleep issue), which seems like a shame, since, in small doses and earlier on in the day, it can have other positive effects (and it's not just caffeine they have come off – they are abiding by 'sleep hygiene' rules like it's a religion... now convinced that there must be something inherently wrong with them because they aren't working).

Some of the 'rules' will have far more influence because they focus on your sleep mechanisms: maintaining a strong sleep drive and the circadian timing of your sleep–wake cycles. Often, though, because they are mixed up among all the other less influential rules and aren't explained very well, the chances of you focusing in on these and doing them with consistency without proper knowledge is low. For example, 'maintain a regular sleep routine' sounds smart and practical, but, just like we learned in Chapter 4, having a fixed bedtime *before* you engage in a consistent fixed get-up time will set you up to fail, and increase your anxiety as you go to bed not sleepy and end up tossing and turning for longer. And who, without understanding the why, is going to start with their get-up time? No one just looking at a standard set of sleep hygiene rules, that's for sure. We will make the easiest moves first, and often those are the ones that will have the smallest impact.

Sleep hygiene rules will do very little in someone with a sleep disorder because sleep disorders are either genetic, very physiological (meaning no amount of behaviour/environment or psychological change will fix it) or, like in the case of long-term insomnia conditions, the new sleep pattern/problem is *so* very ingrained that even influencing the sleep mechanisms and managing expectations/sleep anxiety, which we have focused on with this book, is just the start – a rigorous sleep retraining programme is needed (see the appendix, page 273). Research published in *Sleep Medicine Reviews* found that sleep hygiene interventions had limited impact on improving chronic insomnia, particularly when used as a standalone treatment.

> **The false security of rules**
>
> Sleep hygiene rules give the illusion of control. You think, 'If I follow all the rules, I'll sleep well,' but this is a dangerous oversimplification. If anything, rigid adherence to these rules can make you more anxious about sleep, especially when they don't work. Ever notice how people who sleep well rarely follow sleep hygiene rules? They drink coffee at 8 p.m., scroll Instagram in bed and leave the lights blazing – and yet they sleep just fine. That's because their sleep drive and circadian rhythms are functioning well enough to override minor disruptions.

Let's briefly break down the rules to give you a better understanding:

The important ones

- 🕐 Consistent wake time. This is the most crucial rule. As we've covered in earlier chapters, a consistent get-up time anchors your circadian rhythm and strengthens your sleep drive. Without this, your sleep schedule becomes erratic, no matter how perfect your bedtime routine is.
- 🕐 Morning light exposure. We've seen how natural light in the morning resets your internal clock, signalling to your brain that it's time to be awake. This is especially critical for anyone struggling with sleep–wake timing issues, like jet lag or shift work.
- 🕐 Limiting stimulants close to bedtime. Caffeine and nicotine can delay the onset of sleep by blocking adenosine (the chemical that makes you feel sleepy). But this doesn't mean you need to quit coffee altogether – just aim to avoid it six hours before bed, or accept that for one night maybe your sleep looks a little different.
- 🕐 Managing light in the evening. Light plays a huge role in setting our internal body clock, and the most powerful cue is bright natural light in the morning. That's what helps anchor your circadian rhythm and makes it easier to fall asleep later. But light exposure at night,

especially bright, overhead or long-lasting exposure, can shift your body clock later and slightly suppress melatonin, which may delay sleep in some people. That said, the idea that the blue light from your phone alone is wrecking your sleep is often overstated. The bigger issue is usually what you're doing on the device, the stimulation, scrolling and mental engagement. However, dimming lights and screens one to two hours before bed, and keeping your sleep environment as dark as possible, can still help your brain wind down. Try using low-level lighting in the evening, switch on night mode if you need to use screens and consider blackout blinds or an eye mask if outside light is intrusive.

The 'nice-to-have' ones

These rules might make your sleep environment more comfortable, but they're not game-changers:

- Cool room temperature. Studies suggest that cooler temperatures (around 18°C/65°F) promote deeper sleep. While helpful, this won't fix a chronic sleep problem, or anything that didn't start with your temperature being the problem in the first place!

- Minimizing noise. Noise machines/relaxing sounds can reduce disruptions, but, remember, your brain's RAS is designed to tune out small disturbances if your sleep drive is strong. Also, do bear in mind that the things that can help lull you to sleep might be the very things which stop you from getting into other sleep stages. So, if you do enjoy being 'lulled' to sleep, add a timer at least.
- Comfortable mattress and bedding. Yes, it's nice to have a comfy bed, but this won't solve a sleep disorder like insomnia or a problem that never started with your physical discomfort (and even when it does – why does the bed always get the blame; it could be you need to see a physio for a more ingrained back problem). Plenty of people sleep soundly on lumpy mattresses (just ask anyone who's ever camped). Of course, I'm not encouraging you to sleep on a lumpy mattress – I'm just trying to put things into context.

The overrated ones

- No screens before bed. While the blue wavelengths in light can suppress melatonin production, this rule is often overstated when only talking about screens. If you're using a screen to relax (and not doomscroll), it's not

the end of the world – especially if your get-up time and light exposure are on point. The issue with screens is more the stimulation it brings us, which absolutely impacts what your brain thinks it's time for (not sleeping, that is for sure).
- 🌙 Avoiding meals or exercise in the evening. Digesting a big meal or doing intense exercise close to bedtime can disrupt sleep for some people, but others sleep just fine after both. The key is to know your own body and what works for you – it's very likely you would notice rather quickly if these things had an impact, and that you would course-correct naturally. Adding them as rigid rules to live by to control your sleep will not work.

Rethinking Sleeping Pills: Sedatives, Not a Cure

Sleeping pills are commonly used as a quick fix to 'force' sleep, but they are not a proven solution for sleep disorders, let alone when your problems do not constitute a sleep disorder. In general use, these medications work by sedating you rather than restoring your natural sleep processes. Though I have often heard the term 'reset your sleep' even used by doctors, unfortunately you cannot reset your sleep by knocking yourself out. I think the issue for me with sleeping pills just being used whenever you think you need them is that they create the illusion that any sleep is better than no sleep, even though the quality of that sleep is markedly different from the restorative sleep your body needs. And let's not forget – your body naturally builds a drive in the absence of sleep, and eventually you will sleep again. Often this happens a lot more quickly than expected, but only when this is *not* combined with our sleep anxieties and strange sleep behaviours in a bid to correct the lack of sleep, which will only push sleep away further.

How they work

At their core, sleeping pills induce sedation by enhancing the activity of neurotransmitters like GABA. This action dampens brain activity to help you fall asleep quickly. However, research has shown that the sleep produced by these medications is not the same as natural sleep. For instance, studies using polysomnography have documented that sleeping pills can reduce the amount of slow-wave and REM sleep – both of which, as we've seen, are crucial for physical and mental restoration. In other words, while you may spend more time 'asleep' on a pill, the quality of that sleep is compromised, often leaving you feeling groggy or unrefreshed the next day. Is getting some altered sleep on a sleeping pill better than letting your body figure it out over time?

Research has shown that the sleep produced by these medications is not the same as natural sleep.

Short-term utility versus long-term risk

There are situations when the sedative effect of sleeping pills might be useful. During acute crises – such as the overwhelming stress of grief or a mental health breakdown – your resilience may be so depleted that you need a break from the relentless pressures of the daytime. In these instances, sleeping pills can offer temporary relief by allowing your body to shut down, even if artificially. They provide that necessary pause when your natural ability to wind down is impaired. But I would argue this is only something to consider in exceptional circumstances, and usually a doctor (who needs to prescribe them anyway) will be able to help you make that call.

However, it's important to stress that using sleeping pills as a regular 'sleep hack' is problematic. The sedative effect tricks your mind into believing that forced sleep is a viable substitute for natural, restorative sleep. This can lead to a false sense of security where you think that any sleep is better than none, even if the quality is poor. Over time, this approach prevents you from addressing the underlying behavioural and physiological factors that truly govern healthy sleep, such as maintaining a consistent get-up time and allowing sleep pressure to build naturally. Your body will start to forget how to use those natural sleep processes as you have interjected with something you feel is better. And even if it were, we haven't found a way for you not to get so used to them that they stop working anyway.

One of the most significant risks of habitual sleeping pill use is psychological dependence. When you rely on a pill to induce sleep, you may start believing that you cannot sleep without it. This mindset can erode your confidence in your body's natural ability to regulate sleep. Over time, the thought that 'any sleep is better than no sleep' becomes a crutch – making it difficult to establish healthy sleep habits or trust your own sleep signals.

Moreover, this dependence may mask underlying sleep issues. You might begin to use the pill not just for a one-off crisis, but as a permanent solution, even when the evidence shows that the medication does not improve the quality of sleep. In fact, many users report waking up feeling worse than if they had allowed their sleep to unfold naturally. This altered sleep state may further disrupt your circadian rhythm, creating a cycle that's hard to break.

If you have found yourself buying sleeping pills off the web or trying to find doctors who will prescribe them for you over and over again, it's a really good sign that the beliefs you hold around your sleep are flawed, and you are setting yourself up to fail.

Research published in *BMJ Open* found that regular use of sleeping pills was linked to a higher risk of adverse health outcomes, likely due to their impact on sleep architecture and the development of tolerance. When your body becomes accustomed to artificial sedation, it may require higher doses to achieve the same effect, further deepening the dependency.

Take the case of Laura, a thirty-eight-year-old nurse who turned to sleeping pills during a period of intense personal loss. Initially, the medication helped her 'force' sleep during an emotionally turbulent time. However, as weeks turned into months, Laura noticed that her sleep quality deteriorated. She would fall asleep quickly on the pills, but wake up feeling disoriented and exhausted. The temporary relief turned into a cycle of reliance, and her natural sleep drive diminished as she increasingly depended on the sedative. Eventually, with professional guidance and a focus on rebuilding her sleep habits, Laura managed to wean herself off the pills – realizing that genuine recovery depended on addressing the root causes of her sleep disruption once she was able to do so, rather than continuing the use of the sleeping pills.

Before you reach for a sleeping pill, consider whether you're facing a temporary crisis or a chronic issue that might be better addressed through behavioural sleep strategies. Strengthening your natural sleep routines, managing stress and allowing your body to regulate its own sleep are the key steps towards long-term sleep health. Remember: think before you use, and always be mindful of the true cost of substituting natural sleep with a quick pharmacological fix.

From the sublime to the ridiculous...

In recent years, social media platforms, especially TikTok, have become breeding grounds for a plethora of sleep-related trends. It would be remiss of me not to at least mention these here:

- Cabbage water for sleep. A trend emerged suggesting that drinking boiled cabbage water before bedtime can induce sleepiness. Proponents claim that compounds in cabbage have calming effects. No, just no! There's no scientific evidence supporting this practice, and the taste alone might deter many.

- Mouth-taping. So trendy! This involves taping one's mouth shut during sleep to promote nasal breathing. There is currently no evidence that mouth-taping can improve sleep quality in the average person. There are some very unique cases of mild sleep apnoea that might improve with mouth-taping, but this should be determined and supervised by an experienced associated medical professional. For the average person to limit themselves to nasal breathing takes away a normal biological reflex to open the mouth that happens in certain stages of sleep, helping us to relax and get the most out of that sleep stage. And then, most importantly, having another way to breathe is an evolutionary survival mechanism for when nasal passages are blocked (which you may not necessarily be aware of when awake).

- Bed-rotting. This trend involves spending extended periods in bed, engaging in activities like watching TV or scrolling through phones, under the guise of self-care. Resting is not bad for your body, but ideally you want to spend little time in bed when not sleeping. Keep that association between the bed and 'sleep' strong!

- Sleepy girl mocktail. A concoction of tart cherry juice, magnesium powder and seltzer water, this drink claims to promote better sleep. While tart cherry juice contains melatonin and magnesium plays a role in sleep regulation, the efficacy of this specific combination remains completely unproven.

- Eye-roll sleep hack. This involves rolling one's eyes back repeatedly to induce sleep, based on the idea that it simulates the eye movement during the onset of sleep. Eye movements during sleep are a result of sleep onset, not a cause – trying to force them won't switch your brain off. If anything, focusing on doing this might just make you more alert!

- House tour visualization. A technique where individuals mentally walk through a familiar house, detailing each room to distract the mind and facilitate sleep. While visualization can aid relaxation, it's not impacting those ever-important sleep mechanisms.

- Sleepmaxxing. A trend where individuals go to great lengths to optimize sleep, often involving multiple gadgets, supplements and strict routines. While prioritizing sleep with the other key pillars of health like diet and exercise is important, becoming overly fixated, as this chapter describes, can heavily backfire!

While the allure of quick fixes and novel trends is strong, it's crucial to approach such practices with scepticism.

Many of these trends lack scientific validation and can sometimes do more harm than good. Prioritizing evidence-based sleep behaviours and consulting with healthcare professionals remain the best approaches to achieving restful sleep.

The Psychological Cost of Overloading on Sleep Tools

While sleep tools – whether it's a weighted blanket, a sleep tracker or a cup of chamomile tea – might offer short-term relief, the real issue arises when these tools start becoming central to your sleep routine. The more tools you use, the more you start believing you need them to sleep. This dependency increases anxiety when the tools aren't available and can slowly erode your confidence in your body's natural ability to regulate sleep, leading to a vicious cycle that's hard to break.

When you start relying on external tools, you are, in essence, teaching your brain that sleep cannot happen without them. This is where neuroscience comes into play. Over time, the brain becomes conditioned to associate sleep with a specific tool or action. This is a form of classical conditioning, a psychological process where a neutral stimulus (like a sleep tracker, sound machine or magnesium supplement) becomes linked with the desired outcome (sleep). Once this association is formed, your brain starts to rely on the presence of the stimulus for sleep initiation, even if the tool itself isn't contributing much to the quality of your sleep.

For example, if you begin using a sleep tracker, you may notice that it gives you a score or feedback every morning. Initially, you feel empowered by the data. Over time, however, your brain becomes increasingly reliant on that number, creating a neural pathway where the act of checking your sleep score becomes intertwined with your sense of sleep quality. You start thinking, 'If I didn't get a good score, I didn't sleep well,' even though you might feel perfectly rested. This is the power of cognitive bias, where you allow external feedback to override your internal cues.

Neuroscientifically speaking, this dependency has real consequences. The prefrontal cortex, the part of the brain responsible for decision-making, planning and managing expectations, starts to prioritize these external signals over your body's natural cues. The more you rely on the tool, the less you trust your body's ability to gauge its own needs. This leads to heightened anxiety, which is often referred to as sleep anxiety, and, in turn, this anxiety further impairs sleep quality. Your brain, overwhelmed with thoughts about whether or not the tool will give you the desired result, becomes hyper-aroused, making it harder for you to settle down and fall asleep.

This brings us back to orthosomnia. A 2017 study in the *Journal of Clinical Sleep Medicine* found that participants who excessively monitored their sleep became more anxious and experienced poorer sleep outcomes, even though their actual sleep patterns were normal. The amygdala, a brain region involved in processing fear and anxiety, becomes more active in those who develop orthosomnia, making them more susceptible to stress about their sleep.

When you start using a sleep aid, whether it's a supplement or a gadget, your brain may also release dopamine, the neurotransmitter associated with reward. Initially, this feels great. The act of using a tool becomes rewarding, even if the tool itself doesn't contribute meaningfully to sleep quality. Over time, this can create a dopamine loop, where the brain begins to crave the 'reward' of using the tool, reinforcing the dependency.

The reality check

No tool or supplement will ever replace the foundational sleep habits your brain and body rely on. Tools distract from the real drivers of good sleep: a consistent get-up time, morning light exposure and managing anxiety. It's easier to buy a gadget than to commit to meaningful behavioural change. When you invest time, money and effort into tools, you expect results. And when those results don't come, it reinforces the belief that your sleep is broken, rather than perhaps the tool you are using is flawed. But the most significant and lasting improvements come from strengthening your sleep drive, managing your expectations and aligning your sleep with your body's natural rhythms. As difficult as it may sound, the true solution lies in trusting your body and allowing sleep to happen naturally without an external crutch.

There are a few sleep tools which are quite simple and more aligned with your actual sleep mechanisms – for example, anything that helps you add light to your morning routine, even when natural light is not available. This is because the impact of light has a direct effect on the (circadian) timing of your sleep, which, as you now know, is hugely important to how sleep works.

Before you invest in a sleep tool, ask yourself this: does it directly influence your sleep mechanisms like your circadian rhythm or sleep drive? If the answer is yes, then sure, it might genuinely help over time. If the answer is no, that's okay too. Just be clear about what you're using it for. If it helps you feel calm, relaxed or more at peace, then it's doing something valuable, even if it's not 'fixing' your sleep. That matters.

The key is to manage your expectations. And if you're not getting any benefit at all, not even a sense of calm, then, honestly, don't waste your money.

Breaking the dependency

Have you ever noticed how frustrated you feel when you wake up and check your tracker? Or maybe when you take your magnesium supplement but still wake up exhausted? What does that frustration really cost you – beyond just the hours you've spent trying to make sleep work for you? This cycle of frustration and worry doesn't just affect your mood – it directly impacts your body's ability to relax and enter sleep. The more we invest in these tools, the more we can inadvertently weaken our trust in the one thing we have full control over: our body's ability to sleep naturally. It's time to break that cycle.

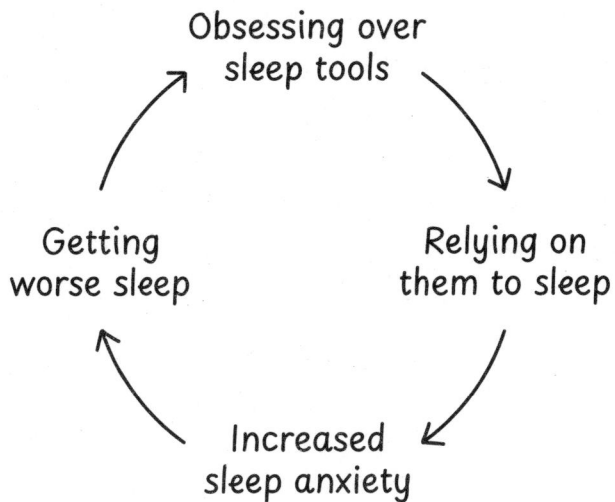

The first step is to reduce your reliance on the tools. This doesn't mean abandoning them altogether, which might fuel anxiety as you go cold turkey, but gradually reintroducing the natural sleep signals your body craves. For example, you could start by setting a consistent get-up time, regardless of how your sleep was tracked. If you use a tracker, shift the focus from the nightly data to long-term trends, avoiding daily fluctuations. If you're using sleep aids like melatonin, consider weaning off them slowly while supporting your sleep with healthy behaviours like morning light exposure and consistent routines.

Ultimately, the key to breaking free from psychological dependency is self-compassion and acceptance of imperfection. Your body is capable of great things, including restful sleep. It just needs the right conditions to thrive. The more you trust your body's natural rhythm and let go of the fear of imperfect sleep, the more you'll find peace with your rest.

We have all felt the weight of a sleepless night – take a deep breath. You're not alone. And you're not broken. This isn't about shaming you for relying on any tools. It's about showing you the path forward, where your own body is the key to rest. You might find this little tool helpful:

The Sleep Pyramid of influence

This pyramid is designed to help you prioritize where to focus your energy (the percentages are for illustrative purposes only and are not evidence-based figures). By addressing foundational issues first and working your way up, you can build a stronger sleep baseline and reduce dependency on external tools or quick fixes. 'The joy of imperfect sleep' sits in the middle because it bridges mindset shifts with practical actions, reminding us that flexibility is essential for long-term sleep health.

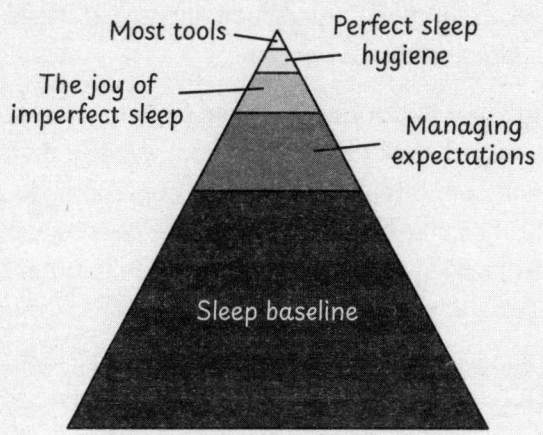

Fixing sleep starts from the bottom – not the top!

1. **Base layer (60 per cent)** – Sleep baseline (sleep drive and circadian rhythm). This is the foundation of good sleep. Strengthening your circadian rhythm and sleep

drive through a consistent get-up time, light exposure and aligning sleep patterns has the greatest influence on sleep quality, duration and timing, and consistent sleep overall.

2. **Second layer (20 per cent)** – Managing sleep expectations and anxiety. Addressing anxiety and setting realistic expectations about sleep reduces stress and fosters a healthier relationship with it, helping you sleep better naturally and stopping you instantly pushing sleep away with your own thoughts!

3. **Third layer (10 per cent)** – The joy of imperfect sleep. Learning to embrace sleep variability and imperfection liberates you from unnecessary stress, making it easier to recover and maintain sleep health. Remember, you will go through natural fluctuations and this is okay! (More on this in Part 3.)

4. **Fourth layer (6 per cent)** – Sleep hygiene (temperature, dark room, and so on). While a dark, cool and comfortable environment contributes to sleep quality, it's far less impactful than the foundation. Use it as a checklist for when you have been through life changes and your habits may have changed.

5. **Fifth layer (4 per cent)** – Sleep tools and supplements (trackers, gadgets, pills, sprays, and so on). These can offer small, incremental improvements – and, for some people, especially those already sleeping well or working on the finer edges of performance (like athletes), that may be enough to feel worthwhile. If you're someone who's curious, data-driven or looking for that final 1–2 per cent gain, tools like trackers

and wearables can be useful. But it's important to remember: they won't fix the root causes of poor sleep. If the fundamentals aren't in place, like a consistent rhythm, healthy sleep drive and manageable anxiety, these tools rarely lead to meaningful or lasting change. In some cases, they can even create more anxiety by over-focusing on metrics that don't tell the full story. If you've already worked on the basics and your sleep is still a struggle, it might be time to speak with a specialist. It could be a sign of an underlying sleep disorder, not something another gadget can solve. That said, there are exceptions: if a tool works with your sleep mechanisms (like using a light box in low-light environments), it may well be part of the solution, not a distraction from it.

Sleep tools are like sprinkles on a cupcake – they can add a little something, but they're not the main ingredient. If you focus on the fundamentals, like building a strong sleep baseline and breaking free from anxiety, you'll see improvements far beyond what any gadget or pill can offer. So, save your money, ditch the pressure and let your body do what it was designed to do. Next time you use some sort of sleep tool, have the right expectations and make sure you enjoy it and that's all it brings you.

PART 3

THE JOY OF IMPERFECT SLEEP

Hopefully, you now understand why we are all fretting so much about sleep. We've given ourselves a reality check and understand how it actually works, we've debunked the most pernicious myths about sleep and we've explored the many mechanisms to help you look after it better. Now we find ourselves here at Part 3, with one more lesson to learn: the goal isn't perfection in sleep – it's freedom. Freedom to sleep without fear. Freedom to wake up after an unusual night and get on with your day. Freedom to trust that your body knows what it's doing.

So, this is a celebration. It's about the joy of sleep as it is – imperfect, adaptive and beautifully resilient. By the end, I want you to feel ready to embody this joy and, most importantly, make peace with your sleep. It was always there for you, you just didn't know it.

CHAPTER 8

The Definition of a Good Sleeper

At this point in the book, you know that measures of what a good sleeper is – for example, a specific duration, a lack of breaks in sleep or feeling euphoric every morning – are probably not really what good sleep looks like. So, how do we define 'good sleep'? Because it looks and feels so physiologically different from person to person, I'm going to use a couple of friends to help me explain what it might look like for you.

Meet Bip. Bip is what we might call a 'stressy sleeper'. Bip tries everything to perfect his sleep. His night-time routine is a checklist of hacks and rituals: noise machine, lavender sprays, 5-HTP supplements, the same bedtime and strict rules about screen time and what he is and isn't allowed to do. If Bip doesn't stick to this, the sleep anxiety gremlins creep in, and Bip believes these rituals are essential for sleep (it makes going away for even just a few nights an absolute nightmare). But Bip still has bad nights – and when that happens, things spiral quickly. Anxiety kicks in, turning the volume up on Bip's temperature and heart rate... and the repetitive thoughts are endless: 'If I fall asleep now, I'll still get five hours. Okay, four hours and forty-five minutes. But what if I don't? I'll be exhausted tomorrow. I won't be able to focus at work. What if this keeps happening?' Bip checks the clock repeatedly, calculating lost sleep and anticipating a terrible next day. He doesn't realize he is pushing sleep and, indeed, a nice rest – the next best thing – further and further away. The next morning, Bip is exhausted, not just from poor sleep, but from the mental strain of worrying.

This pattern repeats. Every bad night feels like proof that something is wrong. Bip spends his days tweaking, troubleshooting and overanalysing his sleep. But the harder he tries, the more elusive sleep becomes. He starts altering his days – less movement and exercise because he believes he doesn't have the energy, and cancelling social events for fear of them affecting his sleep. And while he does all this, his brain is observing this new pattern – more unpredictable time in bed, less movement and fewer activities during the day that bring him happiness – and it's learning it. The brain wants to help Bip get to his goals with ease and so, without Bip realizing it, he's slowly reprogramming his brain onto the insomnia sleep disorder pattern. And he won't stop doing anything he believes makes him sleep, because he has evidence that they work 'sometimes' and that means, if he took them away, his sleep would be so much worse.

Now meet Sally. Sally isn't perfect, but that's the point. She doesn't track her sleep, count her hours or obsess over her bedtime routine. Instead, Sally has a relaxed and trusting relationship with her sleep. Most mornings, she has a consistent get-up time and light/movement routine, and feels ready to start the day. She keeps a consistent sleep opportunity – the time she allocates for rest – but she's flexible and enjoys her rest, even when she's not sleeping. A late night with friends? An extra glass of wine? She knows her body will adapt even if sleep takes a bit of a hit on the night in question. After all, she doesn't do it all the time. When Sally has an unusual night, which looks very different from the usual, she doesn't panic or try to fix it. She doesn't even view it as 'bad' and, while she knows there will be a reason for it, she doesn't spend any time trying to figure out what it was – she just doesn't spend that much time thinking about it. Instead, she carries on, knowing her sleep will recalibrate naturally.

Her morning routine helps her wake up when she's a bit more fatigued, and sometimes she does feel the extra slump during the day, and while she might take it easy on herself, it takes a lot for her to actively change her routine and her mindset to thinking there must be something very wrong. Sometimes, she might spend time away from the bedroom if she's too wired to sleep within her usual sleep opportunity, enjoying a book or quietly watching something she wanted to catch up on, instead of forcing sleep. Even though she doesn't sleep the same all the time, she will describe herself as sleeping well, because she either forgets quickly or just doesn't perceive the unusual nights to be a problem. Most of the time, she feels good and that ratio doesn't really change, unless she's going through something major, at which point she's not really concentrating on what her sleep is doing as she has bigger fish to fry. With this attitude and a fairly consistent sleep baseline that serves her most of the time, she is highly unlikely to develop sleep disorders like insomnia.

Sally's secret? She trusts her body. She embraces sleep as it is – imperfect but resilient. She looks after her sleep consistently but still enjoys herself. She understands that sleep, like other areas of health, is about balance, not perfection.

So here's the question: who do you want to be? You can be Bip, constantly battling sleep, trying to control every detail and feeling defeated when things don't go to plan. Or you can be Sally, trusting in your body's natural processes, embracing flexibility and letting sleep work for you – not against you. The good news is that it's not about perfection. Becoming a Sally isn't about sleeping perfectly every night – it's about letting go of the need to.

The Myth of Perfection: Lessons from Nutrition and Fitness

The pressure to achieve perfect sleep mirrors the pressure we see in other areas of health – particularly nutrition and fitness. And, as with sleep, the pursuit of perfection often does more harm than good.

Take nutrition, for example. The rise of orthorexia – a condition where people become obsessed with eating only 'pure' or 'healthy' foods – shows what happens when the desire to be healthy goes too far. I find this kind of eating disorder very insidious, because it's not obvious to tell physically what's going on – these folk may not look that different to the average person. But the way they control and meticulously measure and analyse what they will and won't eat is beyond obsessive. While prioritizing nutrition is important, becoming rigid and inflexible can lead to social isolation, anxiety and a strained relationship with food and everyone around you. Research shows that an overly restrictive approach to eating can increase stress and reduce overall well-being, even if the food choices themselves are 'healthy'.

Similarly, in the fitness world, chasing perfection often leads to burnout, injury and other health consequences. From the latest CrossFit craze to extreme dieting trends like the Atkins or keto diet, people are constantly searching for the next hack or shortcut – not to use them

The pressure to achieve perfect sleep mirrors the pressure we see in other areas of health – particularly nutrition and fitness. And, as with sleep, the pursuit of perfection often does more harm than good.

as an addition to their well-being practices, but as the sole purpose of their being, and therein lies the problem. Like a cult, there are downsides. The truth is, there are no magic solutions. Science consistently shows that the foundations of health – balanced eating, regular physical activity and sleep – are what matter most. Trying to hack these systems often backfires because our bodies aren't designed to function on extremes.

Sleep is no different. Interestingly, what I notice about patients with chronic insomnia sleep disorder is that they all, to some degree, have sleep anxiety, poor perceptions and beliefs around sleep (which govern their sleep behaviours) or they just don't do any behaviours which influence their sleep mechanisms. I want to know: how rare is it that a sleep problem will remain and turn into insomnia sleep disorder when none of these factors are at play? Even in clients who have chronic illnesses that disrupt sleep, would we be able to diagnose them with insomnia using the classification we have now? I think it would be much less than the current 10–30 per cent of the global population. The fear that sleep will continue to get worse drives our sleep perfection tendencies and we get insomnia anyway.

Perfect is the enemy of good

I can't take credit for this wonderful saying, as it likely comes from the French philosopher Voltaire, who wrote

'Le mieux est l'ennemi du bien', or 'The best is the enemy of the good'. Perfection can prevent us from making progress, achieving good results and just being satisfied with what we have. I can't think of a better way to sum up how to protect and honour your sleep. We have so many examples of how perfection doesn't exist – not in sleep, not in health and not even in the most exact sciences. For the scientifically minded, or if you're just curious about what I might mean, here are some pretty cool examples:

1. Heisenberg's uncertainty principle (quantum physics). At the smallest levels of reality, you can't know both the exact position and speed of a particle at the same time. The harder you try to pin one down, the more elusive the other becomes. Sound familiar? It's like trying to force perfect sleep – the more you chase it, the harder it becomes.
2. Entropy and the second law of thermodynamics (physics). Life naturally moves towards a state of disorder – no system, including the human body or sleep, can maintain perfect order indefinitely. It's normal for sleep to fluctuate, and chasing constant perfection is as futile as trying to stop time.
3. Gödel's incompleteness theorems (mathematics). Even mathematics – the language of logic – has limits. Gödel proved that no logical system can be both complete and consistent. In other words,

there will always be truths that can't be proven within the system. If perfection isn't possible in maths, why should we expect it in sleep?
4. Pi (π) – the infinite number (mathematics). Pi is used everywhere in science, but its exact value can never be fully written down. It's infinite, irrational and impossible to capture perfectly – and yet, we use approximations of it to build bridges, design technology and explore space. Sleep is the same – you don't need perfect sleep to live a healthy, functional life.
5. Imperfect symmetry in nature (physics and biology). This is my favourite. Snowflakes, flowers and even human faces might look symmetrical, but none are perfectly so. Nature thrives on imperfection because that's where beauty and resilience lie. Your sleep doesn't have to be flawless – it just has to be good enough.

Each of these examples is a powerful reminder that perfection is a human invention, not a natural reality. So, if you're holding yourself to impossible standards when it comes to sleep, or anything else, maybe it's time to let yourself off the hook. After all, nature, which is far more powerful than you, can't do it either.

Perfection is a human invention, not a natural reality.

When Sleep Takes a Back Seat – and Why That's Okay

Perfectionism not only creates unnecessary stress, but also ignores the reality that sometimes we need to sacrifice sleep for other priorities – and that's okay. Life is about balance. The goal is to maintain a solid sleep foundation so that when life happens, your body can adapt.

Think about pregnancy. As we've seen, growing a baby often means disrupted sleep – thanks to hormone changes, nausea and the physical discomfort of a growing belly. And yet, women's bodies adapt, continuing to nurture both mother and baby. In fact, lighter broken sleep might not just be a side effect of all the changes; it could be preparing us for what's to come!

Or consider the sleep-deprived days of parenting a newborn. Sleep is fragmented and exhaustion is real, but most parents find a way through, supported by the body's natural resilience. Over time, sleep patterns stabilize, and health returns.

Then there are the sacrifices we choose to make: a late night celebrating a friend's birthday, staying up to watch the sunrise on holiday or taking a red-eye flight to visit loved ones. These moments add richness and joy to life. Yes, they disrupt sleep in the short term, but the body's natural resilience means you can enjoy these experiences without long-term harm.

The key is not to chase perfect sleep every night, but to maintain a consistent baseline. Think of it like a financial budget: if you generally live within your means, an occasional splurge won't break the bank. Similarly, if you prioritize consistent sleep most of the time, your body can handle the occasional disruption.

Everyday sleep anxiety: the stories we tell ourselves

Even when life is calm, many of us fall into patterns of thinking that undermine our sleep:

- 'If I fall asleep now, I'll still get five hours. But what if I don't?'
- 'I didn't sleep well last night, so I can't exercise today – I just don't have the energy.'
- 'I have to get eight hours or I won't function tomorrow.'

These thoughts are common, but they're based on fear, not fact. One or two nights of poor sleep won't ruin your productivity or mood, and even longer-term sleep issues will not be improved with this line of thinking. In fact, research shows that believing you've slept well – even when you haven't – can improve your cognitive performance and mood the next day. This phenomenon, known as placebo sleep, highlights the power of mindset.

Sally understands this. After a rough night, she doesn't dwell on how little sleep she got. She carries on with her day, trusting her body to adjust. If she's tired, she listens to her body – maybe opting for a walk instead of an intense workout – but she doesn't let a bad night derail her. Bip, on the other hand, obsesses over every lost minute of sleep, creating a self-fulfilling cycle of anxiety and exhaustion.

My Bedtime Routine (and Why It Works for Me)

I wanted to include what I do myself for sleep in this book – not because I think my way is the right way or because I want to come across like I've nailed it. Quite the opposite. I want to show you what a real-life sleep routine looks like, even when life is messy.

Here's what I do:

I keep my get-up time the same as much as I can. I get up at 6 a.m. even when sleep has been wonky or I didn't get to bed until late. The time isn't important – everyone's life will dictate something different. It's the consistency. Currently, I'm pregnant, and during the less symptomatic parts, I've been sticking to this, even if I have had to nap during the day. I wanted my body to remember that anchor point, and then I gave myself much grace when I truly needed it by having the odd lie-in. I use a light alarm so I don't have to get up with a noise (irritating!). This is especially wonderful in the winter – when I used to dread getting up. I get out with the dog no matter what – even if I go from a bright get-up environment to a dark winter morning, I will still have plenty of light when I get home and the movement really helps me (besides, the sunrises are later on those dark days and worth getting up for!). It's the anchor point in my day that is important. Sometimes, on the rare occasion, due to life, illness and schedules, I won't be able to do this, but, for the most, I choose to make my life work around this routine which doesn't take up a huge amount of my day.

I do stop my working day fairly consistently and enjoy my evening – staying away from all the stuff that kept my brain active during the day, and then focusing on all the chill stuff that I definitely didn't get time for, like reading and catching up on the latest Netflix series I've been enjoying. My environment will switch from bright and noisy to a little darker and quiet. I'll get ready for bed around the same time most of the time, but I won't take myself to bed until those sleepy cues are calling.

If I wake in the night for longer than a few minutes, and I notice I'm winding up rather than winding down, I'll go back to that evening space. I kind of enjoy it. It's extra time doing some nice chilled things that I don't often get time to do. If I don't get sleepy again for the rest of the night, I'll start my day at the usual time, and transition my environment from the dark and quiet to the bright and alert. Yes, I might be sleepier that day, but my morning habits usually wake me up and keep me going well for most of it.

I do love the sound of rain, so, when I can't wind down in the usual ways, I sometimes put rain noises on a timer because it feels nice and distracts me, and reminds me that resting in that pleasurable state is good.

My sleep has looked different, of course. I got run over and had major surgery so my sleep literally looked like a chronic insomniac's for a while. I'm currently pregnant writing this book, so my night-time will look very different than usual: more wake-ups, more tossing and turning for position (the joys of growing bones). I get sick – I've had Covid way too many times which completely distorted what my sleep looked like for a while – but I can tell you this: my sleep behaviours remained largely the same most of the time (I'd say 80 per cent of the time) and, when I couldn't be resilient because I'm not a robot, my expectations were altered and I could accept fluctuation – besides, that 80 per cent consistency most of the time kept my sleep baseline largely very strong, which meant none of these changes in my life led me on to more chronic sleep issues.

I can't say I track my sleep (other than the kind of experiments we do in the sleep lab testing our kit and training ourselves!), but never say never – if a tool existed to help me manage what I've essentially described in this book, with non-numerical ways to reflect trends over time, I wouldn't necessarily say no if I had a specific goal in mind that I wanted to observe, but the moment it changed my perception or I started relying on it more than my body's own abilities, I would need to stop to avoid spiralling! I, too, would be very much vulnerable to this, even with my experience (after all, I'm only human). I haven't used any sleep tools other than things that help with sleep mechanisms (for example, a light alarm and blackout blinds) and when my environment is largely compromised. If I'm taking a long-distance flight, for example, I will bring an earphone headband (for comfort), so I can listen to rain sounds, and an eye mask to block light.

What matters is that I don't panic when my sleep isn't what I expected. I've built habits that support my sleep enough of the time, so my body can bounce back. I want you to see that you don't need an ideal routine or fancy tools – you just need to understand what works, keep things consistent most of the time and stop chasing perfection.

You don't need to micromanage every detail – your body knows what to do. Embrace flexibility. Life is meant to be lived. Late nights, sometimes early mornings and spontaneous adventures are part of what makes life joyful. Sleep is important, but it's just one part of a bigger picture. So, as you move forward, remember: you don't need perfect sleep. You need good-enough sleep. And

Good news, it's a choice:

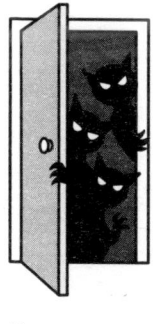 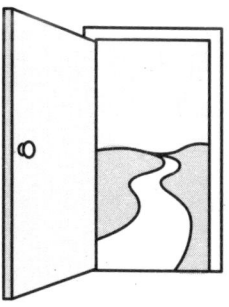

Micromanage your sleep | Think less & work with your sleep

when you trust your body to find that balance, you'll discover a freedom that no sleep hack can offer and find joy in imperfect sleep.

So far, we've let go of the myth of perfect sleep, learned what true evidence-based sleep behaviours look like, embraced flexibility and learned to trust that sleep can bend without breaking. But there's one more shift that can truly change the way you experience your nights and your days, and that's learning to stop blaming sleep for everything that feels off. In the next chapter, we'll look at how to reframe your relationship with sleep itself, so it supports your life instead of running it.

CHAPTER 9

Stop Blaming Sleep for Everything

Imagine this: you wake up after a rough night and instantly brace yourself for a day of fatigue, irritability and poor performance. Sound familiar? If so, you're not alone. Many people blame sleep for their struggles, turning it into a scapegoat for everything that goes wrong. But what if you could break free from this mindset? What if sleep could become your ally instead of your enemy? Let's explore how to reframe your relationship with sleep so that it supports – not sabotages – your life.

It makes me so sad that sleep has become a scapegoat. We blame it for bad moods, low energy, poor performance and even failed relationships. If we sleep well, we expect the day to be perfect. If we don't, we anticipate disaster. This mindset puts unnecessary pressure on sleep, turning it into a perceived enemy rather than the incredible ally it truly is.

In my clinic, I often see clients trapped in this cycle,

such as a recent case where a client's frustration with their fragmented sleep created a cycle of anxiety and hyper-awareness to all the things that they feel went wrong because of their sleep – from being told 'they look tired' to forgetting to pick up the dry cleaning or having a go at their partner. Their focus on every disrupted night amplified their daytime fatigue and changed their behaviour ('I can't do things later in the day in case they impact my sleep'; 'I must rest more to recover and spend more time in bed'; 'I am short-tempered because of my sleep'). While it is true that sleep can impact these things, I do wonder how many of those studies showing these phenomena took into account our readiness to let sleep be the scapegoat, so we didn't have to do uncomfortable things or act in a certain way, especially when the sleep wasn't as broken or 'bad' as we perceived it to be – or might have been in those studies. I am not saying nor did I say to this client that a shift in attitude was going to fix all their sleep issues, but we do know that this attitude makes sleep problems far worse, and that reframing how we think can take away a lot of the stress and anxiety that comes with broken sleep. Let's not forget the power of our own behaviours: when we hold a certain belief – for example, 'sleep is why I look so tired' – we might not do our usual morning routine such as shower, put on our best clothes or make-up, or whatever is involved in our morning routine. We might slump our shoulders and look sad and worried. No wonder people tell us we look tired!

My client's fragmented sleep not only disrupts their nights, but also shapes their attitude and behaviour the next day, which then goes on to disrupt their nights even more. Frustration, self-blame and anxiety fuel this cycle, making restful sleep even more elusive. This emotional response is sometimes referred to as 'sleep frustration syndrome'. Studies show that excessive anger and frustration around sleep create hyperarousal or the sleep sensitivity I described in Chapter 3 – a state of heightened alertness that makes falling asleep and staying asleep even harder. You can't relax into sleep when you're at war with it.

Here's the reality: life is messy, and sleep doesn't control everything. Fatigue, mood and productivity are influenced by countless factors – nutrition, exercise, stress, relationships and mindset, to name a few. Remember how no one ever wants to go to the gym, but when they come out they usually feel much better? Sleep is just one piece of the puzzle. Think back to Sally from the last chapter: I want you to get to a place where you feel like her, rather than just reading about her.

In this chapter, I'll walk you through a practical tool I learned early in my training that will help you shift from frustration to acceptance.

The Sleep Contribution Exercise

The first step is to ask yourself: how much, as a percentage, do you think your sleep contributes to how you feel – physically and mentally – the following day? There are no wrong answers. Some might say 'definitely 90 per cent', while others, after reading this book, might say 'it now feels like 50 per cent'. Whatever your number, draw a circle and colour it in to represent that percentage.

Now, let's pretend sleep doesn't exist for a moment. You have no night-time. You live one long perpetual day. I love doing this because it really makes you think about what sleep and night-time and that break in the day does for us, regardless if you actually sleep during that time or not. Without it, our relationship with time, productivity and even our sense of self would change dramatically. Philosophically, sleep acts as a natural pause – a boundary that separates one day from the next, offering a sense of renewal. Without that boundary, life might feel like an endless continuum, with no natural markers to reflect, reset or recharge.

On a deeper level, sleep shapes how we define productivity and success. In a world without sleep or night-time resting, society might place even greater pressure on constant achievement, stripping away the permission to rest and recharge. This scenario highlights why viewing sleep time as an enemy is so counterproductive – it's not just a biological necessity, but a vital part of what makes us human. By reframing sleep time as an ally, we can embrace its role in helping us navigate the complexities of daily life, rather than resenting it for occasionally falling short of perfection. This is not the entire point of the exercise – I just wanted to point out this other side to sleep which I think is magical and amazing.

Now that sleep doesn't in fact exist anymore, I want you to list all the other things in your life – good or bad – that contribute to how you feel during the day. Note: if you find yourself solely thinking about how sleep affects these things or how they affect your sleep, it's just another example of how much we are consumed by it, in all the wrong ways, and hence why I asked you to imagine it didn't exist. Strip sleep out of the equation completely and think about factors like:

- having a shower
- putting on clothes that make you feel good
- putting on make-up, jewellery or accessories
- looking at your phone first thing in the morning
- whether it's a weekend or a weekday
- walking the dog
- the weather
- noisy neighbours
- food choices
- paying bills
- cold-callers
- watching the sunrise

- someone making you a cup of tea
- exercise
- checking your bank balance
- social time with friends
- arguments with family
- menstrual cycle
- kids, flatmates or partner
- watching the news
- work
- pain
- colour
- smell
- touch
- holidays

Draw a second circle and add these other factors into the new circle, like slices of pie. Add as many as you want. You don't have to be pedantic about the size of each slice, just add them in however you like. Keep going – add them all in no matter how silly or personal they may be. I've had people tell me they couldn't think of anything to write down that affects them – if only that were true! I suspect this is another example of not being able to let go of their beliefs around sleep.

Then, at the very end, add in the contribution your sleep makes. Do you even have enough room? Regardless of what contribution in that pie you can now see your sleep might make (even if you cheated!), this simple tool

List the factors that affect how you feel:

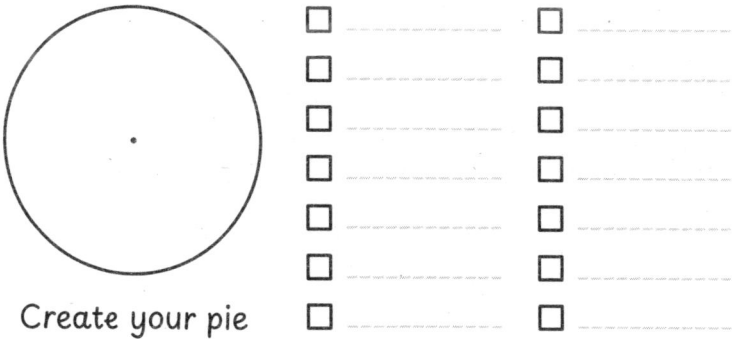

Create your pie

serves as a powerful reminder that sleep isn't responsible for as much as we think. Many factors influence how you feel during the day, and not all of them are within your control. And, even if they are a smaller factor than your sleep, add some of them together and it's a different story.

Now, place a star next to the controllable factors – for example, the weather is not controllable (and yet it often affects us), but how or when you organize your kids' lunchboxes to reduce your manic mornings is.

When you think you're struggling with sleep or your mindset around sleep, revisit this pie chart and remember: your night's sleep is just one slice of the pie. There are plenty of other factors that influence how you feel – and many of them are within your power to change. This shift in perspective is another step towards breaking free from sleep frustration and reclaiming the

What we think contributes to how we feel:

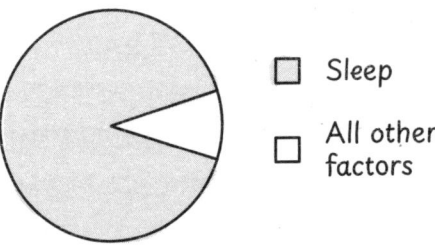

What actually contributes to how we feel:

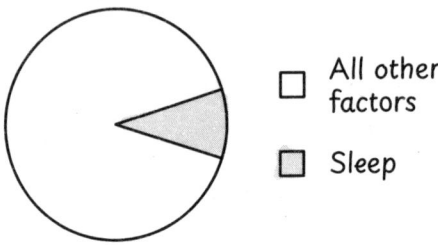

joy of imperfect sleep. And besides, it acts as a bit of a to-do list if you're up at night and want some distractions– planning for the future can be one of them! Keep this pie chart handy, as we move through some other helpful techniques in the next chapter.

CHAPTER 10

Free Yourself from Sleep Perfectionism: How to Be AWAKE

In the last chapter, I used an example that it is so easy to find yourself in – blaming sleep for everything that goes wrong (or right!) with your day when there are so many other variables that affect us. But we need to go further than acknowledging this to get rid of that mindset and stop blaming sleep for everything – we need to prove to ourselves that things can be different.

Sleep perfectionism convinces us that, unless every night is flawless, we've failed. This mindset is exhausting and counterproductive, creating unnecessary stress and unrealistic expectations. Life throws curveballs – chronic illness, menopause, ageing or unpredictable schedules – and these naturally impact sleep. Yet, perfectionism makes us see every disruption as a problem to fix rather than a natural variation to adapt to. And we now know that sleep doesn't need to be perfect to be restorative. By letting go of perfectionism and embracing a balanced approach, you can free yourself from the pressure and start focusing on what really matters: being more awake, present and energized during the day.

The 'How Are You Really?' Scale

In this exercise, I want to demonstrate just how transformative it can be when we shift our focus from the night to the day. So much of sleep anxiety comes from a sense of helplessness – feeling like, once the lights are out, we're at the mercy of our bodies. But what if I told you the real power lies not in the night, but in what you do during the day? This shift is more than just helpful – it's liberating, because we humans crave control, and our waking hours are full of opportunities to take it back. From how we move to how we think, from the routines we create to the way we speak to ourselves, the day is where change begins. And when you start seeing your days as the foundation of your nights, everything shifts. You stop waiting for good sleep to happen to you and start building the kind of life that invites it in, naturally and consistently. That's where the transformation begins.

We need to start with regulating our emotions.

The tendency of many people is to think, 'If I sleep well, I will feel good. If I sleep badly, I will feel awful.' You therefore fall into one of two categories: either feeling good or feeling awful. Sounds a little black

When you start seeing your days as the foundation of your nights, everything shifts.

and white to me – life just isn't this simple. And thank goodness, because it sounds a bit depressing, irrational and unrealistic. It makes sense, from this thinking, that our days are full of self-fulfilling prophecies – 'you look tired' or 'you look great'. I would argue that this usually has more to do with what we did in our morning routine (did we shower, put on nice clothes or a bit of make-up/hair gel?), how we are holding our posture (slumped, dragging feet?) and facial muscles (sad eyes, grimace and frowning?) than it does what night of sleep we had.

It's more helpful to think of how you feel on a spectrum, with feeling good at one end and feeling awful at the other:

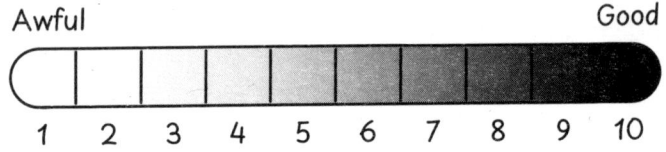

Where are you right now on this spectrum?

Once you really have to think about it, you realize that there have been times when you have felt worse, so you can't be at 0 right now, and times when you have felt better, so you can't be at 10, right? This is a great way of improving how rational and realistic we are about things that affect our feelings which inevitably go on to affect our behaviours, like whether or not we have a shower and wear that nice shirt or the trackie.

Suppose you wake up feeling pretty awful – not the worst you can feel, but really not that great. Suppose you feel only three out of ten. What can you do? You can't be bothered to eat well, so you eat junk food, you don't go for a walk or exercise and you say no to your friend who has invited you out because you don't feel like it. You might spend more time resting than usual. How will you feel by the end of the day? Still a three out of ten, or perhaps even lower than that, maybe a one or a two. Don't assume because you *force* yourself through the day you are any better just because you did the right thing either. This is about your attitude as well. If you're constantly blaming sleep, feeling hard done by or beating yourself up all day, then even if you win the lottery and ride off on a unicorn, your brain will still feel rubbish.

And how well do you think you will sleep after such a day at three out of ten? You see, your thoughts and feelings about your sleep are powerful. They can be even more powerful than the effect of a poor night's sleep ... because they can change your behaviour or impact how your brain thinks things are, even when you should be having the ride of your life!

Suppose, on the other hand, you decide that even though you feel different from usual when you wake up because of an unusual night's sleep, you will make sure that you eat well with intention (I am treating myself!), that you will go for a brisk walk (I can hear the birds sing!) and that you will go out with your friend however you feel (because I always feel better after!). How will you feel by the end of the day? Will it still be three out of ten, or might it go up to six or even seven? Will you sleep better or worse the next night? You have more control than you think!

When you wake up feeling low on the spectrum, revisit the pie chart you created in the last chapter. Instead of thinking, 'I'm going to feel awful all day,' ask yourself, 'Which factors can I control today that will help me move up the spectrum?' Maybe you can't control the weather, but you can decide to wear clothes that make you feel good. You can't control noisy neighbours, but you can still go for a walk to clear your mind. Focusing on what you can do is empowering and helps shift your mindset.

> ### Celebrate small wins
>
> Don't forget to acknowledge your efforts. If you made healthy choices and showed up for yourself, even if you still feel tired, give yourself credit: 'I did my best today, and that matters.' This mindset shift reinforces positive behaviour and improves your long-term relationship with sleep.

So far, we've covered how to stop letting sleep control your day. But what about the nights when sleep actually feels like a problem? What about those times when you're lying awake, fearing the next day, feeling anxious about why you're still awake and slipping back into old habits?

Sleep Won't Always Show Up

The reality is: sleeping poorly is a normal part of life. You don't have to put up with poor sleep every night, but you do have to accept the odd unusual night – or even a few unusual nights – as part of your reality. Even if you were doing everything 'perfectly', life, stress, hormones, illness and completely random factors will affect your sleep.

Wouldn't it be nice if we just didn't care? Because here's the truth: worrying about sleep changes our behaviour, and that behaviour – not the bad sleep itself – can make things worse.

So, how do you stop worrying? Here's a simple blueprint to follow for handling a bad night:

- Start from the right page. If you're panicking over a bad night, tell yourself: for sleep problems to be chronic, they must occur at least three nights a week for three or more months, and for what you're defining as poor sleep to be significantly impacting your life. If this doesn't describe your situation, repeat to yourself: 'This is temporary and quite normal, I am not stuck.' Note: if you do indeed meet these criteria, then do read the sleep disorder appendix for support (see page 273).
- Lean into it. Instead of fighting a bad night, accept it. Your new inner monologue becomes:

'I am not having a usual night for me, and that is okay. I feel a bit funny about it, and that is okay. I am allowed to feel this way. This is normal.'

- Make it fun, make it a luxury – resting is good. Plan enjoyable things for tough nights, such as playing rain sounds, listening to a comforting audiobook or watching your favourite show (while keeping the lights down low). Reward yourself the next day with a small treat. Shift your mindset from 'bad night' to 'bonus time'.
- Relinquish control. If you panic, you may instinctively try to 'fix' your sleep (taking a sleeping pill, cancelling plans, and so on), but this reinforces the fear. Let go of needing control.
- No judgement for reverting to old tricks. Sometimes, you'll slip back into bad habits. That's okay. Behaviour change takes trial and error. If you 'mess up', don't punish yourself – just get back on track.

Repeat. Each time you follow this process, your fear of bad nights will shrink – and, ironically, you'll start having fewer bad nights.

The don't-panic plan for poor sleep

Use the following table to track how your thoughts, actions and mindset shift over time.

Episode	Thoughts Before	Actions During	Thoughts During	Reflections After
Example	I'm away from home – I know I won't sleep well.	I watched TV to distract myself.	I felt anxious but reminded myself this is temporary.	My poor sleep didn't ruin my day as much as I expected!

Each time you go through a tough night, track your experience. Over time, you'll see that your worries about bad sleep start to fade, you will notice not all your experiences are exactly the same and you may see some unhelpful patterns about the way you think which can only be fixed if you notice them!

The AWAKE Mindset

Everything we've covered in this chapter and, indeed, in this book, forms a mindset – one that helps you move through sleep challenges without fear. It's not just a list of tools. It's a way of thinking. And I call it the AWAKE mindset:

A – Accept variation. Sleep doesn't need to be perfect to be powerful. Accepting the natural ebb and flow of your nights – instead of fearing every change – is the first step to freedom. Variation is normal. And it's survivable.

W – Wake up at the same time every day. This is your anchor. Even when the night feels chaotic, your get-up time is the reset button for your brain and body. The earlier you reclaim your rhythm, the faster your sleep recalibrates.

A – Avoid chasing sleep. Trying harder to sleep is like trying harder to sneeze – it backfires. Ditch the clock-watching, the lie-ins and the desperate naps. The less you chase, the faster your body remembers how to find sleep on its own.

K – Keep your daytime strong. Light. Movement. Structure. Boundaries. These are the levers that help regulate your internal systems. When your days are consistent and engaged, your nights follow.

E – Expand your definition of success. Sleep isn't about the perfect score or the deepest stage. It's about how you show up for your life – your energy, your clarity and your mood. Let that be your measure of good sleep.

This isn't about getting a perfect night. It's about learning how to live, thrive and stay grounded – even when sleep is unpredictable. Be AWAKE, not perfect.

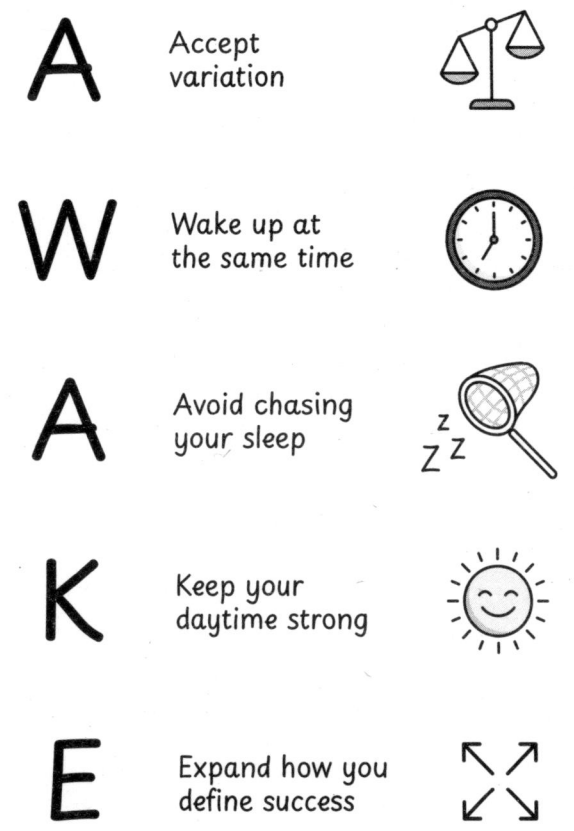

Letting go of sleep perfectionism means accepting both the day and the night as they come. Focus on what you can control during the day, and approach the night with curiosity, not fear. Eventually, bad nights will feel like nothing more than a small inconvenience – and that's when you've truly won the sleep game.

CONCLUSION

Viva La Sleep Revolution!

For twenty years, I've been studying and working with people who feel utterly defeated by their sleep. They're anxious, exhausted and stuck in a cycle of trying everything and still feeling like they're failing. And it's not their fault. Society has done a brilliant job of making us terrified of sleep – of not getting it, of not doing it 'right'. This so often leads to chronic sleep issues, and we do indeed have a global problem with sleep issues right now.

Imagine a world where we did not have this problem. I see this time and time again: when people learn to let go of all the noise and focus on what really matters, their relationship with sleep changes. And when that happens, everything else starts to feel easier, too. Suddenly, enjoying their awake time and experiencing joy is accessible. I see whole families suddenly relax because of one family member finally letting go of the weight they have carried for so long.

This book was never meant to be just another opinion. I didn't write it to join the noise or to take sides in the war on sleep. I wrote it because something had to change. Because the research changed me – not just what I know, but how I live. It made me less afraid. More human. Less obsessed with control, and more in awe of what the body can do when we give it space. And I knew I had to pass that on.

This book was always about balance. Not panic. Not extremes. Not moralizing over what time you go to bed. I wanted to meet you where you are, and walk beside you. Because sleep isn't left or right, good or bad. It's not a virtue or a weakness. It's something we all do. It connects us.

This isn't just about you – it's about the ripple effect of what happens when we stop trying to control sleep and start trusting it. What happens when we shift the narrative – for ourselves, for our kids and for a society that desperately needs to stop blaming sleep for everything.

One client I'll never forget is Rosie, a mum who brought her daughter to see me, completely frazzled because her child wasn't sleeping 'properly'. She had a long list of everything she'd tried: apps, white noise, supplements, even strict schedules. The funny thing? Her daughter was actually fine. She just needed time to grow into her natural sleep rhythms. The real problem was Rosie's anxiety about sleep, which was creating tension at bedtime. It was the first (but not last) time I saw how quickly the impact of how we think about sleep can change a generation. Rosie was just trying to do the right thing, but was on her way to creating a medical disorder in her little one (happily, it only took one session to rectify all this; Rosie was incredibly relieved). And this isn't an isolated case. I've seen it over and over. When adults stress about sleep – whether it's their own or their child's – it creates an environment where sleep feels like a battle. Kids pick up on that tension and start to think there's something wrong, even when there isn't. Then I see their adult selves thirty years later, with chronic insomnia.

Teaching Kids That Bedtime Isn't Scary

We need to talk about how to raise a generation that doesn't grow up fearing sleep or being up at bedtime. If we can break the cycle now, we can stop passing down the idea that sleep is something to be controlled, micromanaged or feared. Children absorb everything we say about sleep, just like they do with food, exercise and emotions and everything else! If they see us panicking over their sleep, they will learn that sleep is something to worry about. If they see us treating a rough night as just a normal part of life, they will learn that sleep is resilient and self-correcting.

How to talk to kids about sleep

When your child wakes up in the night or struggles to fall asleep, they might already be picking up on myths from school, TV or even well-meaning family members. Below are some things they might say and how you can counter them in a positive way:

- 'I didn't get enough sleep, so I won't be able to play well tomorrow!'
  'Actually, your body is really good at making up for sleep when it needs to. You'll still have fun tomorrow, and if you're a little extra tired, your body will just catch up later.'
- 'Why can't I sleep? What if I never fall asleep?'
  'You will. But even if it takes a little while, just resting your body is still good for you. Your brain knows what it's doing, and it will decide when it's ready. You don't have to force it.'
- 'I woke up in the night – is something wrong?'
  'Nope! Everybody wakes up. Grown-ups do it too, we just don't always remember. Your body checks in to make sure everything's okay, and then you go back to sleep when you're ready.'
- 'I had a bad dream. What if I have another one?'
  'Bad dreams are just stories your brain makes up while you sleep. They don't mean anything bad is happening. You don't have to fight them

– just let them pass, and soon a new dream will come along.'

The key is to be reassuring without making a big deal out of sleep. Instead of trying to fix their sleep, we need to help them trust that their body already knows how to sleep. Most importantly for children, we need to make night-time a more magical, relaxing, positive experience, even if they aren't sleeping, not a place where if they are not sleeping, it is scary and lonely.

And, honestly, we need this more than ever. Imagine a generation of kids who grow up unafraid of sleep. Who don't panic about a bad night or feel like they're failing if they don't get a perfect eight hours. Imagine what that could do for their mental and physical health – for the kind of adults they'll become. I would certainly be out of a job!

Letting Go of the Need to Explain Every Sleep Variation

One of the biggest reasons we stress about sleep is that we always want to know why it isn't exactly how we want it to be. We feel more comfortable if we can blame it on something: caffeine, stress, screen time, the temperature, the moon... And yes, some of these things can influence sleep. But the truth is, sleep is far too complex to be reduced to simple cause-and-effect rules.

We all have that moment:

- 'Why did I wake up in the night?'
- 'That coffee after dinner was a mistake; I know my sleep will be bad.'
- 'Why didn't I feel refreshed even though I got eight hours?'

And the honest answer is often: who knows? And does it matter? I spend no time really thinking about any of this when it happens to me, truly. In fact, my poor husband, who as someone who has grown up in our society without studying sleep the way I have, will naturally try to start a conversation with me out of habit about sleep – he will say, 'I feel really tired this morning, I must have had a really bad night's sleep last night' (when I know, especially being pregnant right now and having more breaks in my sleep than him, that he slept normally). I'll counter with, 'Maybe, or maybe it was the fact that you have been stressed with work for the last week, didn't eat properly yesterday and need to hydrate. Anyway, how about we go for a walk in the sunshine?' I remind him that sleep is just one factor, and that what does it matter? We can do a bunch of things that will likely improve his fatigue anyway.

We've also lost something more basic: the ability to sit still and do nothing for even a few minutes. This matters – because sleep isn't instant. It's not supposed to be.

One of the biggest reasons we stress about sleep is that we always want to know why it isn't exactly how we want it to be.

Most people take between fifteen and twenty minutes to fall asleep, and that's completely normal. But because we've become so uncomfortable with any pause – any moment that doesn't produce something, entertain us or feel 'productive' – we start panicking the moment sleep doesn't arrive right away. Instead of waiting it out, we interfere (usually with a phone). It's not the phone that's the problem, it's what the phone represents: escape, stimulation, distraction. What we're really afraid of is stillness. I could write so much about this concept, but, truthfully, a fantastic book has already been written about this in Johann Hari's *Stolen Focus* and I would highly recommend it – it certainly shifted my perspective on doing nothing (and putting down my phone in general).

Your brain knows how to sleep far better than you do. It constantly adapts to stress, hormones, emotions, illness, nutrition, movement, temperature and thousands of other factors you aren't even aware of. Trying to manipulate sleep into perfection is like trying to control your heartbeat – it works best when you leave it alone.

We need to ask ourselves: why do we always need a reason for why our sleep wasn't perfect? Why can't we just accept that sleep – like our energy levels, emotions or appetite – naturally fluctuates?

If we can learn to let go of the constant post-mortem analysis of every bad night, we can finally experience the freedom of trusting that our body already has a plan. Without having to marry a sleep specialist!

Congratulations! You've done the hard work of learning what actually matters when it comes to sleep. You understand that not every piece of sleep advice is worth your time, and a lot of what you've heard previously is either irrelevant or downright harmful. But now, you know better. You've learned:

- How sleep ebbs and flows. How it compensates and looks after you even when it looks different. It's smarter than any hack you could throw at it.
- How to trust your body's natural sleep drive and rhythms. And yes, there are some very influential ways to impact these mechanisms – simple ones.
- Even with all the right information, sleep is not to be micromanaged and perfected. Consistency in your behaviour is key, and then not worrying about the rest!
- That sleep isn't fragile – it's adaptable, resilient and we are lucky to have it. It is not the enemy. It is not at fault for all our problems – it is our best friend, but, like we do sometimes, we are rather demanding of what we think it should provide.

We need to create a world where sleep isn't feared or micromanaged, but celebrated for what it is: a natural, vital part of life that doesn't need fixing. Whether you realize it or not, you're already part of this movement. By learning to trust your sleep, you're shifting the way you think – and that shift doesn't stop with you. When you talk to your friends about what you've learned, when you challenge the myths you hear, when you show your kids that sleep isn't something to stress about, you're leading the way.

This isn't about being perfect. It's about showing up with what you've learned and being open to sharing it, if you want to, because it would really help us all. Here's how you can keep the momentum going:

- Talk about it. Share your experience with others. Whether it's a friend, a colleague or a parent at the school gates, tell them what you've learned. Explain why sleep doesn't need to be perfect and how small, consistent changes can make a big difference.
- Challenge myths. When someone says they need eight hours every night or that they're doomed after a bad one, gently push back. Share what you now know – that sleep is resilient, adaptable and so much more forgiving than we've been taught.
- Model it for your kids. Show your children that sleep isn't scary or fragile. Let them see you trusting your body, embracing variability and not sweating the bad nights.

You've done the work for yourself. Now you have the chance to spread that change to others – to your family, your friends and even to the next generation. Together, we can create a world where sleep isn't an enemy, but an ally. A world where we trust rest, embrace imperfection and give ourselves the grace to let sleep do what it does best.

Forget about sleep. Focus on being AWAKE!

APPENDIX

Medical Sleep Disorders: When You Need More Support

While my goal throughout this book has been to help you shift your mindset around sleep and develop a healthier, more trusting relationship with it, for some of you, the challenge may go beyond variability, habits and perspective. If you've applied the key principles of this book over time – embracing sleep's natural rhythms, maintaining consistent influential habits and letting go of control – but your sleep is still persistently poor and not serving you, it may be time to consider whether an underlying sleep disorder is at play (and, even if you have a known medical disorder that can impact sleep, it is still worth considering if there is something else going on). Don't ignore it.

This book itself can act as a screening tool. If you feel that your sleep mindset is solid and your lifestyle supports good sleep, but nothing seems to work, then it's more evidence for your medical team to investigate further, and this section is for you. To note here: sometimes it's hard to *apply* the concepts in this book because, for example, the anxiety is too high and it's become stressful or you just find some of the more pragmatic advice really hard to stick to, like your body just won't let you do it. Don't ignore this either – beyond us just finding something a bit cumbersome or tough, not being able to find a way to adapt these concepts to your body and lifestyle often means support is needed, so do not ignore this; help is out there.

Many sleep disorders remain undiagnosed for years because sleep disturbances are often dismissed as lifestyle issues, stress-related or simply 'part of getting older'. Even within the medical field, basic sleep education is shockingly lacking – resulting in patients being told to 'just get to bed earlier' or 'reduce stress' rather than receiving real help. Sleep disorders are often primary conditions, meaning they exist independently of other health problems, even if they may be triggered or worsened by life events and other conditions.

I do appreciate that it's incredibly hard to get diagnosed and treated in sleep medicine unless you suffer from a common sleep disorder that the doctor has seen before, but my point here is that the more you know about the process, what you can screen yourself for and understand, the more likely it is you can present in such a way that you will be listened to, or you will find it far easier seeking out the appropriate clinics and support for you. When I started re:sleep, my insomnia programme, it was to do exactly this – bring the support to the client, because so often in this area we get ignored. re:sleep is an accessible online tool for those suffering from the most common sleep disorder, insomnia.

In this section, I'll break down the most common sleep disorders:

- chronic insomnia disorder
- obstructive sleep apnoea
- restless legs syndrome
- circadian rhythm disorders
- parasomnias (night terrors, sleepwalking, REM behaviour disorder, and so on)

For each, I'll explain what I think might help you get some support:

- The textbook definition (how it's typically described in medical literature and what your doctor is thinking).
- How it actually presents in real people (what it looks and feels like in day-to-day life – because

sometimes it's different, and the way you describe it to your doctor might be different. It's worth knowing what they need to hear, and how it might feel for you).
- When to seek help (because waiting years isn't the answer – but knowing how, where and when to look is helpful).

If anything in this section resonates with you, please seek specialist advice. Sleep disorders are treatable, but only if we acknowledge them in the first place.

Chronic Insomnia Disorder

The textbook definition

Insomnia is the persistent difficulty in falling asleep, staying asleep or waking too early at least three times per week for three months or longer, despite having the opportunity to sleep. It significantly impacts daytime function (mood, energy, concentration, and so on).

How it presents in real life

This is not just 'struggling with sleep'. People with chronic insomnia feel utterly isolated and broken, often hearing unhelpful remarks like: 'I don't know what's wrong with you – I just hit the pillow and I'm out!' Saying this to an insomniac is like asking someone with depression, 'Why can't you just be happy?' It's dismissive, ignorant and it prevents real support from happening.

Insomnia isn't just one thing – it can be a mix of:

- sleep sensitivity (the more sleep becomes broken, the more sensitive you become to the environment such as noise or pain, making sleeping harder, like a vicious cycle)
- lack of sleep drive (not generating enough sleep pressure – making it harder to fall asleep and stay asleep)
- a dysregulated sleep pattern (poor body clock alignment – now you're feeling awake during the night and tired during the day, and your body only reinforces this once it becomes a bit of a pattern)
- poor misconceptions and ideas about sleep (which have a direct impact on what behaviours you choose to alter it – often the wrong ones)
- sleep anxiety (the less you have/the more broken it is, the more you worry, and the more you worry, the worse it gets…)
- other health conditions impacting sleep (pain, hormonal shifts, chronic health conditions, mental health issues, and so on)
- reduced sleep depth – suddenly sleep always feels light and unrefreshing (a mixture of a lot of the other factors coming into play here)

There are more factors, but my point here is they are all usually going on at once, so it makes sense that a lot of stuff on the market won't help or will only give you short-term improvements – they simply don't target them all, and therefore fail in the long run. At re:sleep, we call them the 'seven horsemen' because of how powerful they are. We also notice that because of how much people think they have tried to fix their insomnia, they feel very untrusting of anything that promises to solve it. Those other useless hacks and chemical concoctions have made them feel like there is something wrong with them because they didn't work for them – when it was simply the wrong tool for the job. It is not you – effective treatments are available. I promise!

You might have noticed this book does cover some of these factors, because knowing that some can turn into insomnia helps you *avoid* chronic insomnia, but if the book hasn't helped or has only taken you so far, it's likely this faulty programming has been going on for some time. Instead of just reading something useful, you likely need medical intervention. I know sometimes your sleep may not present the way other chronic insomnia presents, but if it's been going on for a while now and the other conditions below can't explain it, it's likely you need to accept that it is a type of insomnia.

When to seek help

If your sleep problems have lasted longer than three months, are affecting your quality of life and are not improved by lifestyle changes, or indeed this book, you need targeted treatment – and it exists, contrary to how untrusting you feel after trying all that other stuff.

Specialists use the insomnia severity index on the next page to assess symptoms of insomnia, which you might find useful when discussing your own symptoms with your medical healthcare provider.

Treatment: The gold standard is cognitive behavioural therapy for insomnia (CBT-I). This is *not* 'sleep hygiene' as you know it and as we have discussed it in the book. It's an evidence-based programme that retrains your brain to undo insomnia. Think of it like losing weight or quitting smoking – it's challenging but completely doable with the right support. It takes a few weeks, or months if you want to do it slower depending on what you can manage, but it is absolutely life-changing when you give it proper attention. Sometimes, medication is prescribed to help you manage the condition, but, unfortunately, there is no evidence as of yet that it can rid you of the problem for good.

I spend most of my time now at my online platform re:sleep and during my own consulting at Sleepyhead Clinic helping people with exactly this – undoing years of damaging sleep patterns. If you've made it through this

Insomnia Severity Index (ISI)

Subject ID: _____   Date: ____

For each question below, please circle the number corresponding most accurately to your sleep patterns in the LAST MONTH.

For the first three questions, please rate the SEVERITY of your sleep difficulties.

1. Difficulty falling asleep:

None	Mild	Moderate	Severe	Very Severe
0	1	2	3	4

2. Difficulty staying asleep:

None	Mild	Moderate	Severe	Very Severe
0	1	2	3	4

3. Problem waking up too early in the morning:

None	Mild	Moderate	Severe	Very Severe
0	1	2	3	4

4. How SATISFIED/dissatisfied are you with your current sleep pattern?

Very Satisfied	Satisfied	Neutral	Dissatisfied	Very Dissatisfied
0	1	2	3	4

5. To what extent do you consider your sleep problem to INTERFERE with your daily functioning (e.g., daytime fatigue, ability to function at work/daily chores, concentration, memory, mood).

Not at all Interfering	A Little Interfering	Somewhat Interfering	Much Intefering	Very Much Interfering
0	1	2	3	4

6. How NOTICEABLE to others do you think your sleeping problem is in terms of impairing the quality of your life?

Not at all Noticeable	A little Noticeable	Somewhat Noticeable	Much Noticeable	Very Much Noticeable
0	1	2	3	4

7. How WORRIED/distressed are you about your current sleep problem?

Not at all	A little	Somewhat	Much	Very Much
0	1	2	3	4

Guidelines for Scoring/Interpretation:
Add scores for all seven items =
Total score ranges from 0-28

0–7	=	No clinically significant insomnia
8–14	=	Subthreshold insomnia
15–21	=	Clinical insomnia (moderate severity)
22–28	=	Clinical insomnia (severe)

book, you're already better prepared for sleep retraining than most, because you understand the why. Now, it's about taking the next step.

It's unlikely you need a sleep study to 'rule in' insomnia – a good medical history usually suffices – so don't let anyone hook you into expensive sleep studies (especially if you're paying!) without a good alternative reason, such as ruling out another sleep disorder.

Obstructive Sleep Apnoea (OSA)

The textbook definition

OSA is a sleep disorder where breathing repeatedly stops and starts due to the airway becoming narrowed during sleep. Symptoms include loud snoring, choking or gasping at night, and excessive daytime sleepiness. It's more common in overweight individuals, because there is extra pressure around the neck area. There are other types of apnoea, but this is the most common one we see.

How it presents in real life

Many people with sleep apnoea don't even know they have it. They think they sleep just fine but feel exhausted every day – often needing to nap to compensate. In some cases, the sleepiness during the day won't be so prolific, but that's unusual. It is often flagged if you have a partner, who is more concerned as they notice the constant sleepiness, grumpiness (because who isn't when they are constantly needing to sleep!), strange noises coming from you at night and a constant fear of you not breathing again, not to mention the snoring can get very loud!

Sleep apnoea isn't just an annoyance; it's a risk if left untreated. It's linked to high blood pressure, heart disease, diabetes and even an increased risk of stroke. What's important to note is you won't just stop breathing and die in your sleep – this event is very rare and not usually because someone has untreated sleep apnoea.

When to seek help

If you:
- snore loudly or your partner notices you stop breathing in your sleep
- wake up with headaches or a dry mouth
- feel exhausted even after more than seven hours of sleep
- struggle to stay awake during the day

Another symptom can be frequently going to the toilet to pass urine in the night. So, if, more often than not, you get up twice or more on a regular basis, don't ignore it when you see these other symptoms as well. The following 'STOP-Bang' questionnaire can also be helpful to determine if you are at risk: http://www.stopbang.ca/osa/screening.php.

If you feel excessively sleepy during the day so that you need to nap regularly despite good sleeping hours at night, you should absolutely speak to your GP. It is not normal and, once you get on that treatment pathway, there are always ways to make improvements. But instead, people live with it: they're often told, 'You're just lazy' or, 'You need to go to bed earlier.' Somehow we seem to have labelled people who fall asleep in inappropriate situations regularly like meetings, driving or talking to someone as lazy or rude. It makes no sense – I can be lazy and rude and I don't seem to suffer regularly from the ability to fall asleep at the drop of a hat. Most of these people have tried to get more sleep, but the problem persists. Make sure you insist on sleep studies in this case – these kinds of disorders often get ignored for other medical issues or for your own poor habits. Narcolepsy, for example, takes an average of eleven years just to get diagnosed, and this is one of the most common signs (but it itself is not common, hence why I haven't gone into more detail here regarding this, but should sleep apnoea be ruled out in investigation, it is worth exploring this disorder or other excessive sleepiness issues further).

The Epworth Sleepiness Scale (ESS) is a useful tool for excessive daytime sleepiness:

https://www.asthmaandlung.org.uk/conditions/obstructive-sleep-apnoea-osa/epworth-sleepiness-scale.

Treatment: A respiratory sleep study or oximetry sleep study can confirm OSA, and CPAP therapy (a device that keeps your airway open) is highly effective and the gold standard treatment. There is a lot of work out there on trying to create other methods of resolving the issue, but, at the time of writing, nothing can make it go away like CPAP in most cases. In some people, merely losing weight can reduce the OSA to the point where the sleepiness and medical risks are dramatically lowered, but I do find in a lot of clients I have seen, to have the motivation to lose that weight, even CPAP in the short term, in order to improve how you feel and your energy levels during the day, can be very handy.

Restless Legs Syndrome (RLS)

The textbook definition

RLS is a neurological disorder causing an uncontrollable urge to move the legs, especially at night/in the evenings. It tends to delay sleep and breaks it up as you find yourself tossing and turning.

How it presents in real life

It feels like crawling, tingling or aching in the legs that only stops when you move. People describe it as 'pure torture' – it sabotages their ability to relax and can make sleep impossible. It can lead to chronic insomnia. It can be common to see in pregnancy.

When to seek help

If you experience the following very regularly and it's causing sleep to become elusive:
- an urge to move your legs in the evening or before bed
- sleep disruption due to leg movements

Treatment: Because the cause of RLS can be tricky to determine, blood tests are very useful and then, depending on the cause, various medications or supplements, such as iron (if iron deficiency is observed – and this is one of the most common causes in pregnancy) can be very helpful. Even if it's tricky to determine the cause, behavioural adjustments to sleep, similar to CBT-I for insomnia, can improve symptoms.

Circadian Rhythm Disorders

The textbook definition

These are disorders where the body's internal clock is misaligned with the external world, such as delayed sleep phase syndrome (DSPS). This can look like a tendency to fall asleep very late (for example, 3 a.m.) and then your sleep running into the day (for example, midday) with little natural ability to regulate it so that it fits in better with your lifestyle. Circadian rhythm disorders are genetic, and go beyond our lifestyles being responsible – it feels very hard for someone with this kind of genetic condition to simply 'do all the right things' and sleep to just flip to a more normal schedule. You can also have advanced sleep phase syndrome (ASPS) which has the opposite sleep pattern to this, and various others such as free running disorder (where the sleep period gets later and later each day). In general, while the quality of sleep can be affected in these cases, the real difference between this type of sleep and the average person's sleep is the *timing*.

How it presents in real life

- Night owls who can't fall asleep before 2–4 a.m., even if exhausted.
- People who wake up hours too early and can't get back to sleep, and generally need to go to bed very early as well.
- Shift workers struggling with constant sleep deprivation.
- No routine at all, no matter what you do – almost like the sleep schedule is different every night.

It's important to note that this is not the same as insomnia, where the sleep is very broken or lacking, but, if you can get it, it tends to happen between our usual night-time hours. These circadian conditions often just look like sleep is running and sometimes very well, but the schedule is all over the place.

When to seek help

In circadian rhythm disorders, feeling awake during the hours that everyone else seems to feel awake to manage relationships or hold down a job, for example, seems quite impossible unless you can adapt your entire life to it. Sometimes I see people who have managed this, but, in most cases, it is incredibly difficult to do. Seek help if your body clock is preventing you from functioning in daily life.

Treatment: Strategic bright-light exposure, melatonin timing and behavioural therapy can retrain your circadian rhythm. Detailed sleep studies are funnily enough not that helpful. Less complex monitoring over longer periods of time, such as several weeks of monitoring movement with a sleep diary and/or actigraphy (a movement sensor), can be far more helpful at trying to figure out what 'schedule' your biological clock seems to be entrained to.

Parasomnias (Sleepwalking, Night Terrors, and So On)

The textbook definition

Parasomnias are unusual behaviours during sleep, such as sleepwalking, night terrors or acting out dreams. It can be more specific – like having sex in sleep, being aggressive in sleep or sleep eating. There are many and so what I have outlined here is just the most common.

How it presents in real life

- Waking up screaming but not remembering why.
- Walking or talking in sleep without awareness.
- Physically acting out dreams.

When to seek help

If your safety is at risk (for example, falling out of bed or leaving the house while asleep), or somebody else's is, or there are other symptoms alongside it, such as daytime symptoms of significant sleepiness or significant distress during the day, it's important to seek help. If you find symptoms manageable, then there is no need to seek support – as we talk about in the book, lower frequency of parasomnias can be normal in some people and the practices in the book can help when these types get exacerbated.

Treatment: It depends on the type of parasomnia, but improving sleep stability helps significantly. Sleep studies can help, especially with identifying type which leads to specific treatment, but sometimes a good medical history is all that's needed. Medication can be helpful (and, on that note, some medication can increase the likelihood of them, so it's important to check with your GP what could be impacting your sleep). This is where trying to pinpoint where in your sleep this is happening and getting more detail through a study can be helpful. Alcohol, sedatives (like sleeping pills) and stimulants (including caffeine) can worsen parasomnias by disrupting natural sleep patterns and increasing abnormal arousals.

While I've outlined the more common and overarching themes of sleep disorders and what you might look out for, bear in mind that there are over eighty recognized sleep disorders according to the *International Classification of Sleep Disorders*, so if you're unsure you fit into these categories but sleep is still a problem, please speak to a doctor. In any case, make sure you outline what you have already done and tried, to show that your mindset is balanced about your sleep and that you try to take care of your sleep mechanisms in the most influential ways possible. This is to avoid them asking you to do these things (or just throwing sleep hygiene advice at you). You should not be ignored if you can provide that kind of evidence.

If you see yourself in these descriptions, please don't ignore it. These conditions are not personality flaws – they are medical conditions that deserve real treatment. And treatment can be life-changing.

Lastly, when looking for support, which I know can feel a bit sparse (but understanding your condition better can be very helpful in your search), you need to make sure you see the right specialist. Sleep specialists are just like other medical specialists – they cover a broad area as there are so many fields of sleep medicine. You wouldn't see a knee surgeon who specializes in knee replacements for older people with arthritis if you are in your twenties and suffered a football injury – there are sports injury specialist knee surgeons who may be better suited. Similarly, you want to check the qualifications *and experience* of a sleep specialist to make sure they are right for you. A good sleep specialist will always recommend the most appropriate care for you, even if it is not them, and be able to demonstrate why that might be.

Notes and References

Introduction

p. 4 **Take the often-cited Penn State study, which looked at a very specific group: people with chronic insomnia *and* objectively measured short sleep duration** Vgontzas, A. N., Liao, D., Bixler, E. O., Chrousos, G. P., and Vela-Bueno, A., 2010. Insomnia with short sleep duration and mortality: The Penn State cohort. *Sleep*, *33*(9), pp. 1159–64.

p. 6 **according to one of the most recent analyses, we are currently between 10 and 30 per cent of the global population** Mai, E., and Buysse, D. J., 2008. Insomnia: Prevalence, impact, pathogenesis, differential diagnosis, and evaluation. *Sleep Medicine Clinics*, *3*(2), pp. 167–74.

Chapter 1

p. 14 **Historical and anthropological evidence suggests that many pre-industrial societies slept in alignment with natural light** Yetish, G., et al., 2015. Natural sleep and its seasonal variations in three pre-industrial societies. *Current Biology*, *25*(21), pp. 2862–8.

p. 14   **In medieval Europe, for example, records describe this biphasic sleep, where people naturally slept in two phases** Ekirch, A. R., 2001. Sleep we have lost: Pre-industrial slumber in the British Isles. *The American Historical Review, 106*(2), pp. 343–86.

p. 15   **Anthropological studies of modern hunter-gatherer societies** Yetish, G., et al. Natural sleep and its seasonal variations in three pre-industrial societies.

p. 15   **when people fell short, they began to feel inadequate (as demonstrated by researcher Kohler in his study on sleep tracking, and many others)** Kohler, M., Barth, J., and Stoll, M., 2016. The effects of self-monitoring and technology on sleep quality and sleep anxiety. *Journal of Sleep Research, 25*(2), pp. 154–60.

p. 19   **writer Jessa Gamble (in *The Siesta and the Midnight Sun*) describes anthropological observations from circumpolar cultures** Gamble, J., 2011. *The Siesta and the Midnight Sun: How Our Bodies Experience Time.* Goose Lane Editions.

p. 20   **Surprisingly, modern data shows that national averages for sleep duration don't vary as wildly as you'd expect** Marqueze, E. C., et al., 2015. Natural light exposure, sleep and depression among day workers and shiftworkers at Arctic and equatorial latitudes. *PLOS One, 10*(4), p. e0122078.

p. 31 **When researchers and military organizations realized that the body could adapt its sleep architecture** Caldwell, J. A., and Caldwell, J. L., 2005. Fatigue in military aviation: An overview of US military-approved pharmacological countermeasures. *Aviation, Space, and Environmental Medicine*, 76(7 Suppl), pp. C39–51.

p. 37 **research shows that even a one-hour shift can temporarily affect sleep and mood** Kantermann, T., Juda, M., Merrow, M., and Roenneberg, T., 2007. The human circadian clock's seasonal adjustment is disrupted by daylight saving time. *Current Biology*, 17(22), pp. 1996–2000.

p. 37 **One study found that our internal clocks don't shift as fast as the social clock does** Wittmann, M., Dinich, J., Merrow, M., and Roenneberg, T., 2006. Social jetlag: Misalignment of biological and social time. *Chronobiology International*, 23(1–2), pp. 497–509.

p. 38 **some studies show a small uptick in cardiovascular events right after the shift** Janszky, I., and Ljung, R., 2008. Shifts to and from daylight saving time and incidence of myocardial infarction. *The New England Journal of Medicine*, 359(18), pp. 1966–8.

p. 42 **research confirms that this is when sleep becomes more fragmented** Mindell, J. A., Cook, R. A., and Nikolovski,

J., 2015. Sleep patterns and sleep disturbances across pregnancy. *Sleep Medicine*, 16(4), pp. 483–8.

p. 49 **even if they start the process of building a stronger sleep baseline during menopause, there are still significant gains to be had** Young, T., Rabago, D., Zgierska, A., Austin, D., and Finn, L., 2003. Objective and subjective sleep quality in premenopausal, perimenopausal, and postmenopausal women in the Wisconsin Sleep Cohort Study. *Sleep*, 26(6), pp. 667–72.

p. 53 **some research suggests they might spend less time in deep sleep and more time in lighter, less restorative sleep** Cortese, S., Faraone, S. V., Konofal, E., and Lecendreux, M., 2009. Sleep in children with attention-deficit/hyperactivity disorder: Meta-analysis of subjective and objective studies. *Journal of the American Academy of Child & Adolescent Psychiatry*, 48(9), pp. 894–908.

p. 53 **Some research also suggests that autistic people produce melatonin differently** Tordjman, S., et al., 2013. Advances in the research of melatonin in autism spectrum disorders: Literature review and new perspectives. *International Journal of Molecular Sciences*, 14(10), pp. 20508–42.

p. 55 **there's evidence that the way the brain cycles through sleep in these conditions may be altered** Kishi,

A., et al., 2011. Sleep-stage dynamics in patients with chronic fatigue syndrome with or without fibromyalgia. *Sleep*, *34*(11), pp. 1551–60.

Chapter 2

p. 59 **The electroencephalogram (EEG) showed sleep was an active process** Berger, H., 1929. Über das Elektrenkephalogramm des Menschen. *Archiv für Psychiatrie und Nervenkrankheiten*, *87*(1), pp. 527–70.

p. 59 **Then REM sleep was discovered, showing that sleep is anything but passive** Aserinsky, E., and Kleitman, N., 1953. Regularly occurring periods of eye motility, and concomitant phenomena, during sleep. *Science*, *118*(3062), pp. 273–4.

p. 60 **But it wasn't until the 1950s and 60s, through human isolation experiments (where people lived in caves for weeks), that we confirmed humans have their own built-in clock, too** Aschoff, J., and Wever, R., 1962. Spontaneous rest-activity cycles in relation to the light-dark cycle. *Proceedings of the National Academy of Sciences*, *48*(4), pp. 696–701.

p. 65 **The Penn State cohort studies on sleep and mortality found that significantly higher mortality risk was associated with people who had both short sleep duration and poor-quality, unrefreshing sleep** Vgontzas,

A. N., et al. Insomnia with short sleep duration and mortality: The Penn State cohort.

p. 65 **An umbrella review in *Frontiers in Medicine* found that poor sleep quality amplifies the health risks of short sleep** Gao, C., et al., 2022. Sleep duration/quality with health outcomes: An umbrella review of meta-analyses of prospective studies. *Frontiers in Medicine*, 8, p. 813943.

p. 65 **another meta-analysis found that long sleep durations – often assumed to be healthier – were also linked to increased mortality** Cappuccio, F. P., D'Elia, L., Strazzullo, P., and Miller, M. A., 2010. Sleep duration and all-cause mortality: A systematic review and meta-analysis of prospective studies. *Sleep*, 33(5), pp. 585–92.

p. 66 **In fact, polysomnography (gold standard sleep studies) consistently shows that people with insomnia, for example, often sleep much more than they think they do** Harvey, A. G., and Tang, N.K.Y., 2012. (Mis)perception of sleep in insomnia: A puzzle and a resolution. *Psychological Bulletin*, 138(1), pp. 77–101.

p. 67 **Large-scale genetic and population studies show huge individual variability in sleep need** Dashti, H. S., et al., 2019. Genome-wide association study identifies genetic loci for self-reported habitual sleep duration supported by accelerometer-derived estimates. *Nature Communications*, *10*(1), p. 1100.

p. 69 **Indeed, in the research, we see that even when a tracker deliberately lies about your sleep data being bad, it will drive poor health outcomes during the day** Shusterman, A., Bar, M., and Baror, L., 2022. False feedback from sleep trackers negatively affects cognitive performance and subjective well-being. *Journal of Sleep Research*, *31*(6), p. e13723.

p. 70 **coined by research teams looking at the effects of things like sleep tracking** Baron, K. G., Abbott, S., Jao, N., Manalo, N., and Mullen, R., 2017. Orthosomnia: Are some patients taking the quantified self too far? *Journal of Clinical Sleep Medicine*, *13*(2), pp. 351–4.

Chapter 3

p. 79 **There's robust research to support this** Fortier-Brochu, É., Beaulieu-Bonneau, S., Ivers, H., and Morin, C. M., 2012. Insomnia and daytime cognitive performance: A meta-analysis. *Sleep Medicine Reviews*, *16*(1), pp. 83–94.

p. 82 **Surveys of educational providers show that sleep medicine is one of the most under-taught areas during medical training** Mindell, J. A., and Bartle, A., 2008. Sleep education in medical school curriculum: A national survey of

U.S. medical schools. *Sleep*, *31*(7), pp. 825–8; Romiszewski, S., et al., 2020. Medical student education in sleep and its disorders is still meagre 20 years on: A cross-sectional survey of UK undergraduate medical education. *Journal of Sleep Research*, *29*(6), p. e12980.

p. 83 **Based on hundreds of clients I've worked with (and much research!), the solution lies in what I like to call 'reverse-engineering sleep'** Furukawa, T. A., et al., 2024. Components and delivery formats of cognitive behavioral therapy for chronic insomnia in adults: A systematic review and component network meta-analysis. *JAMA Psychiatry*, *81*(2), p. 123.

Chapter 4

p. 90 **Studies show that spending too much time in bed can actually lead to 'sleep fragmentation'** Spielman, A. J., Saskin, P., and Thorpy, M. J., 1987. Treatment of chronic insomnia by restriction of time in bed. *Sleep*, *10*(1), pp. 45–56.

p. 94 **Studies indicate that unwinding before bed can reduce levels of the stress hormone, cortisol** Backhaus, J., Junghanns, K., and Hohagen, F., 2004. Sleep disturbances are associated with increased evening cortisol concentrations in primary insomnia. *Journal of Psychosomatic Research*, *58*(2), pp. 115–22.

p. 112 **Research suggests that sudden auditory alarms can activate the sympathetic nervous system** Tassi, P., and Muzet, A., 2000. Sleep inertia. *Sleep Medicine Reviews*, 4(4), pp. 341–53.

p. 118 **According to research, people with consistent wake times across the week tend to report higher sleep quality and are significantly less likely to experience symptoms of insomnia** Bei, B., Wiley, J. F., Trinder, J., and Manber, R., 2016. Beyond the mean: A systematic review on the correlates of daily intraindividual variability of sleep/wake patterns. *Sleep Medicine Reviews*, 28, pp. 108–24.

Chapter 5

p. 126 **Psychologist Kenneth Lichstein and others have described this as a kind of *insomnia identity*** Lichstein, K. L., 2017. Insomnia identity. *Behaviour Research and Therapy*, 97, pp. 230–41.

p. 129 **Research published in the *Journal of Psychosomatic Research* found that individuals who experienced objectively poor sleep but didn't perceive it as a problem were less likely to experience the negative health outcomes often associated with insomnia** Fernández-Mendoza, J., et al., 2011. Cognitive-emotional hyperarousal and subjective insomnia: A matter of perception. *Journal of Psychosomatic Research*, 70(4), pp. 314–21.

p. 131 **there's some research suggesting that short-term sleep deprivation can reduce overthinking and inhibition** Tempesta, D., et al., 2010. Lack of sleep affects the evaluation of emotional stimuli. *Brain Research Bulletin*, 82(1–2), pp. 104–8.

p. 132 **In another fascinating study from the *Journal of Clinical Sleep Medicine*, researchers found that people with high levels of 'sleep reactivity' (a term for how much stress about sleep impacts their lives) were more likely to develop chronic insomnia** Drake, C. L., Pillai, V., and Roth, T., 2014. Stress and sleep reactivity: A prospective investigation of the stress-diathesis model of insomnia. *Journal of Clinical Sleep Medicine*, 10(9), pp. 989–96.

Chapter 7

p. 163 **It's no coincidence that the global sleep aids market was valued at over $70 billion in 2024** Precedence Research, 13 Dec. 2024. Sleep aids market size, share, and trends 2024 to 2034. Retrieved from https://www.precedenceresearch.com/sleep-aids-market [accessed 15 May 2025].

p. 165 **But studies show they're less than 50 per cent accurate at identifying these stages compared to polysomnography** de Zambotti, M., et al. Wearable sleep technology in clinical and research settings. *Medicine & Science in Sports & Exercise*, 51(7), pp. 1538–57.

p. 166 **a study published in *Sleep Health* found that sleep trackers often overestimate total sleep time and underestimate how often you wake up during the night** Chinoy, E. D., et al., 2021. Performance of seven consumer sleep-tracking devices compared with polysomnography. *Sleep Health*, 7(3), pp. 261–7.

p. 166 **when we manipulate the tracker results in studies to show poor sleep – even when it's been good – the health outcomes are much the same as someone who did indeed sleep poorly** Draganich, C., and Erdal, K., 2014. Placebo sleep affects cognitive functioning. *Journal of Experimental Psychology: Learning, Memory, and Cognition*, 40(3), pp. 857–64.

p. 168 **A 2017 study in *Journal of Clinical Sleep Medicine* documented cases of orthosomnia caused by sleep trackers** Baron, K. G., et al. Orthosomnia: are some patients taking the quantified self too far?

p. 173 **One review found that magnesium supplements may help older adults with insomnia, but the effects were**

mild at best Mah, J., and Pitre, T., 2021. Oral magnesium supplementation for insomnia in older adults: a systematic review and meta-analysis. *BMC Complementary Medicine and Therapies*, 21(1), p. 125.

p. 176 **A meta-analysis found that melatonin improved sleep onset by an average of seven minutes** Ferracioli-Oda, E., Qawasmi, A., and Bloch, M. H., 2013. Meta-analysis: Melatonin for the treatment of primary sleep disorders. *PLOS One*, 8(5), p. e63773.

p. 177 **The most common evidence-based side effects of melatonin are daytime drowsiness, vivid dreams or nightmares, dizziness, headaches and gastrointestinal discomfort** Besag, F. M. C., Vasey, M. J., Lao, K. S. J., and Wong, I. C. K., 2019. Adverse events associated with melatonin for the treatment of primary or secondary sleep disorders: A systematic review. *CNS Drugs*, 33(12), pp. 1167–86.

p. 177 **A review in *Sleep Medicine Reviews* found valerian to be 'possibly effective'** Fernández-San-Martín, M. I., et al., 2010. Effectiveness of valerian on insomnia: A meta-analysis of randomized placebo-controlled trials. *Sleep Medicine*, 11(6), pp. 505–11.

p. 179 **one systematic review highlighted that many studies reporting improvements in insomnia symptoms had significant limitations** Suraev, A. S., et al., 2020.

Cannabinoid therapies in the management of sleep disorders: A systematic review of preclinical and clinical studies. *Sleep Medicine Reviews*, 53, p. 101339.

p. 181 there's some science to show that they can indeed have a subjective, positive effect on some people (those with anxiety-related psychiatric disorders) Ekholm, B., Spulber, S., and Adler, M., 2020. A randomized controlled study of weighted chain blankets for insomnia in psychiatric disorders. *Journal of Clinical Sleep Medicine*, 16(9), pp. 1567–77.

p. 183 A study in the *Journal of Caring Sciences* found that white noise improved sleep in patients surrounded by constant noise in a coronary care unit Farokhnezhad Afshar, P., Bahramnezhad, F., Asgari, P., and Shiri, M., 2016. The effect of white noise on sleep quality in patients admitted to a coronary care unit: A randomized controlled trial. *Journal of Caring Sciences*, 5(2), pp. 103–11.

p. 183 A study in *Frontiers in Human Neuroscience* found that pink noise enhanced slow-wave sleep and memory in older adults Papalambros, N. A., et al., 2017. Acoustic enhancement of sleep slow oscillations and concomitant memory improvement in older adults. *Frontiers in Human Neuroscience*, 11, p. 109.

p. 189 A small but widely cited study found that transcranial direct current stimulation during sleep

enhanced slow-wave activity and improved memory consolidation in participants Marshall, L., Helgadóttir, H., Mölle, M., and Born, J., 2006. Boosting slow oscillations during sleep potentiates memory. *Nature*, *444*(7119), pp. 610–13.

p. 189 **Another study in *Frontiers in Human Neuroscience* showed that timed auditory stimulation (like pink noise) could increase slow-wave activity during sleep in some participants** Papalambros, N. A., et al. Acoustic enhancement of sleep slow oscillations and concomitant memory improvement in older adults.

p. 195 **The origins of this phenomenon started when the term was coined in 1977 by American psychiatrist Peter Hauri** Hauri, P., 1977. *Current Concepts: The Sleep Disorders*. Upjohn.

p. 197 **Research published in *Sleep Medicine Reviews* found that sleep hygiene interventions had limited impact on improving chronic insomnia, particularly when used as a standalone treatment** van Straten, A., et al., 2018. Cognitive and behavioral therapies in the treatment of insomnia: A meta-analysis. *Sleep Medicine Reviews*, *38*, pp. 3–16.

p. 199 **Studies suggest that cooler temperatures (around 18°C/65°F) promote deeper sleep** Okamoto-Mizuno, K., and Mizuno, K., 2012. Effects of thermal environment on sleep and circadian rhythm. *Journal of Physiological Anthropology*, 31(1), p. 14.

p. 199 **this won't fix a chronic sleep problem, or anything that didn't start with your temperature being the problem in the first place** van den Heuvel, C. J., Ferguson, S. A., Dawson, D., and Gilbert, S. S., 2005. Effect of mild manipulations of core body temperature on sleep onset latency. *European Journal of Applied Physiology*, 94(3), pp. 273–8.

p. 202 **However, research has shown that the sleep produced by these medications is not the same as natural sleep** Buysse, D. J., 2013. Insomnia. *JAMA*, 309(7), pp. 706–16.

p. 202 **For instance, studies using polysomnography have documented that sleeping pills can reduce the amount of slow-wave and REM sleep** Roehrs, T., and Roth, T., 2010. Drug-related sleep stage changes: Functional significance and clinical relevance. *Sleep Medicine Clinics*, 5(4), pp. 559–70.

p. 205 **Research published in *BMJ Open* found that regular use of sleeping pills was linked to a higher risk of adverse health outcomes** Kripke, D. F., Langer, R. D., and Kline, L. E., 2012. Hypnotics' association with mortality or cancer: A matched cohort study. *BMJ Open*, 2(1), p. e000850.

p. 211 **A 2017 study in the *Journal of Clinical Sleep Medicine* found that participants who excessively monitored their sleep became more anxious and experienced poorer sleep outcomes, even though their actual sleep patterns were normal** Baron, K. G., et al. Orthosomnia: are some patients taking the quantified self too far?

Chapter 8

p. 227 **Research shows that an overly restrictive approach to eating can increase stress and reduce overall well-being** Dunn, T. M., and Bratman, S., 2016. On orthorexia nervosa: A review of the literature and proposed diagnostic criteria. *Eating Behaviors*, 21, pp. 11–17.

p. 233 **In fact, lighter broken sleep might not just be a side effect of all the changes; it could be preparing us for what's to come!** Mindell, J. A., et al. Sleep patterns and sleep disturbances across pregnancy.

p. 234 **In fact, research shows that believing you've slept well – even when you haven't – can improve your cognitive performance and mood the next day** Draganich, C., and Erdal, K. Placebo sleep affects cognitive functioning.

Chapter 9

p. 243 Studies show that excessive anger and frustration around sleep create hyperarousal or the sleep sensitivity I described in Chapter 3 Espie, C. A., Broomfield, N. M., MacMahon, K. M., Macphee, L. M., and Taylor, L. M., 2006. The attention–intention–effort pathway in the development of psychophysiologic insomnia: A theoretical review. *Sleep Medicine Reviews, 10*(4), pp. 215–45.

Chapter 11

p. 268 I could write so much about this concept, but, truthfully, a fantastic book has already been written about this Hari, J., 2022. *Stolen Focus: Why You Can't Pay Attention – and How to Think Deeply Again.* Crown Publishing Group.

Appendix

p. 279 Specialists use the following insomnia severity index to assess symptoms of insomnia Morin, C. M., 1993. *Insomnia Severity Index (ISI)* [Database record]. APA PsycTests.

Acknowledgements

To the lovely team at Atlantic Books, and to Drummond Moir in particular. Thank you for seeing something in me right from the beginning. For believing that the world was ready for a book that challenged the norm. For trusting me to share a message that could feel bold and disruptive, but needed to be said.

To all the international publishers who chose to bring this book into their part of the world. Thank you for your faith in me and for sharing the belief that the sleep conversation needs to change. I am so grateful that this story, this mission, can travel across borders and cultures.

To my incredible assistant, Lydia, thank you for keeping everything running while my head was buried in writing and research. Your calmness, organization and support behind the scenes made it possible for me to actually finish this book. I truly couldn't have done it without you!

To my beautiful baby boy, Ander. You were growing in my tummy while I wrote every chapter. You reminded me every day to be humble and grounded. Pregnancy sleep is no joke, and you made sure I stayed connected to the very people this book is for. I hope your generation grows up never feeling like they have to earn their sleep or be perfect to deserve rest.

To my husband, Tom. There are not enough words. You are my biggest fan and the most constant support I could ask for. You looked after me so patiently and lovingly while I was pregnant and writing. You listened to me go back and forth on ideas a million times without ever rolling your eyes. And most importantly, you made me belly laugh every day. There is no better life elixir than that.

To Pasco. You are my shadow and you never complained when I sat for hours typing, waiting patiently for walks, pats and treats. And to Pawel, my purry little friend who constantly reminded me to make sure the book was saved somewhere other than my laptop, as you walk across the keyboard several times a day.

To the friends and family who stuck by me even when I had my head down for months on end. Thank you for your patience when I disappeared. For your support when I resurfaced. And for never making me feel guilty about following dreams that often took me far away from what it means to be a convenient friend or an available relative. I noticed. And I'm grateful.

To every person who has ever shared their sleep story with me. Whether in clinic, in a message, in one of my programmes, or face to face. You are the reason this book exists. Your trust, honesty and vulnerability inspired every page. Thank you for letting me in. You have taught me more than you know.

And to anyone reading this who has ever felt like they're failing at sleep. I hope this book helps you let go. I hope it shows you that you are not broken, you do not need fixing, and you certainly do not need to fear your nights. This is your permission slip to stop overthinking and start trusting yourself again. Sleep does not have to be perfect to be powerful.

Ready to put this into practice?

Get better sleep in two weeks with Stephanie's BBC Maestro online course.